Recognising, Understanding and Treating Nameless States

In this captivating volume, Bernd Nissen considers the multiplicity of nameless states, and the impact of their discovery on psychoanalytic theory and practice.

The nameless is considered through a variety of lenses: trauma, unrepresented states, autistoid/autistic states, breakdown, non-existence, and unrepressed/unstructured consciousness. Nissen draws upon the work of Freud and Bion to inform his exploration of nameless states and the ways in which they might be located, understood and conceptualised. He illuminates the processes of transformation into the psychic and asks how nameless states can be psychically anchored. Clinical vignettes are used throughout to illustrate the consequences for treatment, as well as interpretations of complex holding situations.

This book will be of interest to analysts both in practice and in training, as well as psychotherapists and mental health practitioners wishing to understand nameless states more deeply.

Bernd Nissen is a training and control analyst, and a psychoanalyst (DPV/IPV) in private practice in Germany. His main areas of work are autistoid disorders, psychoanalytic technique, and scientific and theoretical questions on psychoanalysis. He has edited and published several journal articles and books in various languages.

The Routledge Wilfred R. Bion Studies Book Series
Series Editor: Howard B. Levine, MD

The contributions of Wilfred Bion are among the most cited in the analytic literature. Their appeal lies not only in their content and explanatory value, but in their generative potential. Although Bion's training and many of his clinical instincts were deeply rooted in the classical tradition of Melanie Klein, his ideas have a potentially universal appeal. Rather than emphasising a particular psychic content (e.g. Oedipal conflicts in need of resolution; splits that needed to be healed; preconceived transferences that must be allowed to form and flourish, etc.), he tried to help open and prepare the mind of the analyst (without memory, desire or theoretical preconception) for the encounter with the patient.

Bion's formulations of group mentality and the psychotic and non-psychotic portions of the mind, his theory of thinking and emphasis on facing and articulating the truth of one's existence so that one might truly learn first hand from one's own experience, his description of psychic development (alpha function and container/contained) and his exploration of **O** are "non-denominational" concepts that defy relegation to a particular school or orientation of psychoanalysis. Consequently, his ideas have taken root in many places…. and those ideas continue to inform many different branches of psychoanalytic inquiry and interest.[1]

It is with this heritage and its promise for the future developments of psychoanalysis in mind that we present *The Routledge Wilfred Bion Studies Book Series*. This series gathers together under newly emerging and continually evolving contributions to psychoanalytic thinking that rest upon Bion's foundational texts and explore and extend the implications of his thought. For a full list of titles in the series, please visit the Routledge website at: https://www.routledge.com/The-Routledge-Wilfred-Bion-Studies-Book-Series/book-series/RWBSBS

Howard B. Levine, MD
Series Editor

---

1 Levine, H.B. and Civitarese, G. (2016). Editors' Preface, *The W.R. Bion Tradition*, Levine and Civitarese, eds., London: Karnac 2016, p. xxi.

Recognising, Understanding and Treating Nameless States

A Psychoanalytic Exploration

Bernd Nissen

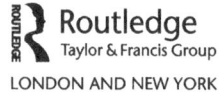
Routledge
Taylor & Francis Group

LONDON AND NEW YORK

Designed cover image: Getty / s-cphoto

First published 2024
by Routledge
4 Park Square, Milton Park, Abingdon, Oxon OX14 4RN

and by Routledge
605 Third Avenue, New York, NY 10158

Routledge is an imprint of the Taylor & Francis Group, an informa business

British Library Cataloguing-in-Publication Data
A catalogue record for this book is available from the British Library

Library of Congress Cataloging-in-Publication Data
Names: Nissen, Bernd, 1959– author.
Title: Recognising, understanding and treating nameless states:
a psychoanalytic exploration / Bernd Nissen.
Other titles: Routledge Wilfred Bion studies book series.
Description: Abingdon, Oxon; New York, NY: Routledge, 2024. |
Series: Routledge Wilfred Bion studies book series |
Includes bibliographical references and index.
Identifiers: LCCN 2023032079 (print) | LCCN 2023032080 (ebook) |
ISBN 9781032561660 (paperback) | ISBN 9781032561691 (hardback) |
ISBN 9781003434207 (ebook)
Subjects: MESH: Psychoanalytic Theory | Psychotherapeutic Processes |
Psychoanalytic Therapy | Unconscious, Psychology |
Psychological Trauma | Autistic Disorder
Classification: LCC RC506 (print) | LCC RC506 (ebook) |
NLM WM 460.2 | DDC 616.89/17—dc23/eng/20230929
LC record available at https://lccn.loc.gov/2023032079
LC ebook record available at https://lccn.loc.gov/2023032080

ISBN: 978-1-032-56169-1 (hbk)
ISBN: 978-1-032-56166-0 (pbk)
ISBN: 978-1-003-43420-7 (ebk)

DOI: 10.4324/9781003434207

Typeset in Times New Roman
by codeMantra

Contents

Preface, which can also be a conclusion[1]

The nameless is nothing.

The nameless has many names, e.g. non-existence, breakdown, autistic/autistoid disorders, early traumas, unrepresented states, unrepressed unconscious, etc., but is unknown.

The nameless is not sensual in essence, not even pleasure/unpleasure, pleasure and pain apply.

The nameless is not psychic.

The nameless is not psychic because the psychic arises in relationship and is grounded in the sensual.

The nameless has fallen out of relationship; the hope of relationship has been abandoned.

The nameless is not conscious and not unconscious.

The nameless is entropic, maelstrom of silent, dark dissolution.

The nameless cannot be expelled.

The nameless generates pulsating excitations in its environment.

The nameless must be encapsulated. Envelopments form around these encapsulations, which cause pleasure/unpleasure, attraction and repulsion.

The nameless in its entropic power leads to the excitations of these sheaths being perverted, that is, sought for their own sake.

The nameless therefore remains covertly virulent; autistoid measures are used to further shield it.

The nameless can be indirectly noticed by the Pcpt-Cs via the actual excitations of the perverse-autistoid mechanisms.

The nameless can be sensed in its existence via the performance of the Pcpt-Cs, thus finding its way into the relationship.

The nameless needs a relationship to become.

The nameless can then occur for the self and the object in the relationship (moment of presence).

The nameless can receive a presentative name in the sublation.

The nameless can become from a name (conception) to a thought and finally be used.

This book tries to circle these sentences from different perspectives and to present them metapsychologically, theoretically, treatment-technically and above all clinically. It can therefore only be an attempt.

At the centre (Chapter 2) is the moment in which the nameless occurs, the presence moment. The nameless is silent and hidden – only the perverse-autistoid sheaths can be very loud and intrusive. But "at some point" it can be intuitively sensed in free-floating attention, the central method of psychoanalysis. Analysand and analyst sense that "something" is coming towards the couple. In this run-up to the coming event, specific treatment techniques become relevant that are oriented towards the sensual and co-experiencing. This is because the basal sensual residues, grouped around pleasure and unpleasure, offer the first starting point and make encounter possible. Sensual and experience-oriented interventions are heard in the transference and create hope for an understanding object. The complementary structures that emerge lay the foundation for the nameless to happen and be named in the relationship. The presence moment is not conscious, not unconscious, qualityless, yet there in the Pcpt-Cs for the couple. It must be sublated into the presentative, i.e. the incomprehensible complexity must be bound in a name. The presentative is itself so complex that it can never be completely decomposed discursively. The name is a discovery, a creation and a subjugation of the couple.

But the sublation into a name, into a conception, and its use succeeds for the self initially only in the presence of the object. The presentative is only the beginning of becoming, which can be understood as the attempt to gain (partial) sovereignty over entropy. The presentative must be transformed into a thought (i.e., into a representation) that survives the absence of the object. This process can become very turbulent, as the object cannot be distinguished from the early traumatising one. Violent, aporetic dynamics can arise in which suicidal, psychotic and psychosomatic processes can occur. They represent a benign progression, but in statu nascendi they cannot be distinguished from malignant, threatening regressions. If this transformative process succeeds, a thought can arise, thus the apparatus for thinking the nameless. Then processes can follow in which separation and dependence are worked out through the use of the object.

From this perspective, the moment of presence is not a singular, isolated event, but is embedded in preceding and subsequent processes. These processes are complicated, complex, risky and without certainty in vivo. The presence moment is the central node, but without the preceding processes it would not only not happen, but would simply remain undeterminable. Even more important are the subsequent processes up to the formation of thoughts. If they are absent or fail in the treatment, the conception disintegrates. Even the absence of object use can still have a problematic effect.

In addition to these basic theoretical and theoretical determinations, an attempt will be made to examine methodical, methodological and treatment-technically dimensions associated with the nameless (Chapter 3). The focus here is on considerations of sensual sensations, sensualisation, psychicisation and psychic stabilisation, i.e. possibilities of transforming nameless states. The further developments resulting from Bion's theory are discussed in detail. It is argued that these methods and techniques, i.e. α-function, reverie, dreaming, hallucinosis, intuition, are specific sub-groupings and forms of free-floating attention. They are important extensions and make it possible to encircle, divine and understand the nameless. Postbionian interpretations and further developments are critically discussed.

Chapter 4 attempts to connect these conceptualisations and considerations with selected aspects of psychoanalytic theory and practice. The starting point regarding the sensual is re-examined. The analytical attitude that the sensual requires is that of holding, the holding function. Since the sensual qualities are not differentiated, proceeding only according to pleasure-unpleasure, the careful differentiation in holding is particularly important, since in this way, first, the sensual experience differentiates itself, or rather blank presentations can become sensual, and, second, the analyst can emerge as an object in the psychoanalytic sense. The hope that arises in the patient is thus founded in two ways: He develops a psychic function, regredience, for the nameless realms, and experiences a holding, patient object that offers him sensual qualities without becoming determinative. The aporetic complexity of these processes is discussed in a detailed example.

Chapter 1 provides a detailed overview of the different approaches to conceptualising the nameless in a broader sense. The historical beginnings in Bion, Winnicott and also Meltzer are pointed out, then the enormous developments following Tustin in the study of disorders from the autistic/autistoid spectrum are detailed. The work in French psychoanalysis, which developed in isolation from the studies of autistic dynamics, revolves around other phenomena, but these are complementary and compatible with the considerations of autistic/autistoid states: The white series, the clinic of the negative and regredience explore voids in the psychic and how they can be "filled." Contemporary conceptualisations of "unrepresented states" or the "non-repressed unconscious" take up many aspects of the aforementioned work, but assume that these states are located in the non-repressed unconscious. But can states that are not conscious and not unconscious be located in the unconscious? This question is discussed again in Chapter 4.

In the short, in the final chapter (Chapter 5) there is a critique of Bion's concepts, especially the α-function and the infinite. The view that one function should operate in all psychic systems clashes with the Freudian view that different functions operate in individual systems. The Freudian view allows for a more differentiated and deeper investigation of the psychic apparatus, especially for binocular processing in Cs/Pcs and Ucs. The concept of the infinite, which Bion introduces and to which Matte-Blanco gives a central position, is also too indeterminate and is based on a set-theoretical conception of the psychic, which is nevertheless to be doubted.

The question arises whether it is not time to put aside the ladder of Bionian conceptualisations with which we have climbed into unknown realms....

Berlin, December 2022

Note

1 In the book, the generic masculine is used for better readability.

Nameless states

The concept of the nameless is an embarrassment – an embarrassment, however, that has existed in psychoanalysis for a long time and encompasses a field of phenomena that has many names. Nameless states lie beyond (?) or this side (?) of the repressed unconscious or even the psychised.

DOI: 10.4324/9781003434207-1

Chapter 1

Psychoanalytical considerations on nameless states

1.1 Beyond the repressed unconscious?

In my opinion, Freud probably suspected all his life that there are psychoanalytically relevant areas beyond the repressed unconscious. Reminder: "Everything that is repressed must remain unconscious; but let us state at the very outset that the repressed does not cover everything that is unconscious. The unconscious has the wider compass: the repressed is a part of the unconscious" (Freud, 1915e, 166).

But what does that mean? Is only the repressed unconscious the accessible part of the unconscious via derivatives? Is the unconscious beyond the repressed the non-accessible part of the psychic system? Can complexes of the wider unconscious be psychic ones that have not yet acquired meaning? Are there psychic complexes that have not yet acquired meaning, or is meaning the characteristic of the psychic in the reference system of the psychic? Are the methods developed for the repressed not suitable for exploring the non-repressed unconscious? Does it escape all influence? Do Matte-Blanco's investigations of the infinite, symmetrical unconscious refer to the non-repressed unconscious? Where are non-psychicised states to be located? In the wider unconscious? In the Interpretation of Dreams, Freud postulated that "the unconscious is the true psychical reality" (Freud, 1900a, 613). Can the non-psychicised then be found in the psychic systems Cs, Pcs and Ucs, e.g. in the extended Ucs.

For Freud, non-psychicised states do not seem to have been unthinkable. The question whether seduction is real-traumatic or phantasised could be relevant here. But apart from this, he had held throughout his life to the concept of actual neurosis as a disorder whose origin is not to be found in infantile conflicts. It was Baranger, Baranger and Mom (1988) who determined the actual as the purely traumatic, thus making this disorder one from the non-psychisised spectrum. But also his speculations on perversion in relation to neurosis ("neurosis as negative of perversion," 1905d), on narcissistic neuroses (psychoses), herein also his first descriptions of symbolic equation (1915e, 299), point in the direction beyond neurosis. Freud stated impressively clearly that in very early childhood there are events that are inscribed but cannot be remembered, but are acted out (1914g, 149f). With his sensing that the shadow in melancholia has something threateningly permanently

DOI: 10.4324/9781003434207-2

present, cannot really be grasped objectally (1917e), he went a step further: He sensed that there is something quite different in melancholy than in depression, as described by Abraham (1916–17), for example, in his theory of regression. Freud uses the image of the two-dimensional shadow, that is, a threat that is literally intangible. A deeper understanding of the shadow has, in my opinion, only been formed in the last decades and was related to nameless states (s. Nissen, 2016; see Roussillon, 2015, who associates the shadow with the negative). Then it was especially the work on the concept of trauma (1916–17, 1920g, 1926d) and the discovery that there is a "Beyond the Pleasure Principle" (1920g), herein a repetition-compulsion that goes beyond acting out, and the postulation of a death drive that opened the door to new subject areas of psychoanalysis, even if Freud could not investigate them. Finally, it is worth mentioning the work "The Ego and the Id," in which the first topical model was replaced/supplemented by the second one, with which uncertainties in the concept of the systemic Ucs seem to be overcome, but from which then also emerged discoveries that, on a completely different level, transformed the concepts of the unconscious, preconscious and conscious. E.g. in the concept of splitting of the Ego (1927e, 1940e), I think, a primary-process-like activity is outlined that, with our current understanding, is neither conscious nor unconscious. It lets something be there, which is not unconscious, but is not really systemically consciously grasped either.

The title "Beyond the Pleasure Principle" could be programmatic. The pleasure principle is the central feature of the unconscious. If there is a beyond of the pleasure principle, could this also mean that there is a beyond of the unconscious? Then Freud would have sensed three subject areas: the repressed neurotic, the psychotic and one beyond the unconscious, one that is not yet psychically represented, perhaps at its core neither psychically conscious nor unconscious. If the first two areas, neurosis and psychosis, are explored clinically and theoretically in psychoanalysis for decades, we seem to be only slowly recognising the outlines of the third area, which has been studied more and more for the last 50 years and has become established in the last 20–25 years.

1.2   The discovery of nameless states

At the beginning of the 1970s, several psychoanalysts observed similar phenomena that lay beyond psychic representation. In my opinion, besides Winnicott with his reflections on breakdown (1974; see below) and Meltzer et al. (1975), with investigations on autism, herein two-dimensionality, adhesive identifications, dismantling, etc., it was above all Bion who postulated "a domain of the non-existent" (Bion, 1970, 20):

I have not come across any realization that corresponds to such a state though I can imagine a stupor so intense that it might seem to do so... Some patients with whom I am familiar achieve a state, to which I wish to apply the term "non-existence", for a few moments at most; this is followed by an externalization or evacuation of "non-existence". "Non-existence" immediately becomes an object that is immensely hostile and filled with murderous envy towards the quality or function of existence wherever it is to be found.

(Bion, 1970, 20)[1]

Bion remains committed to Kleinian thinking here; for the unbearable state of non-existence is evacuated and felt as "immensely hostile and filled with murderous envy towards the quality or function of existence wherever it is to be found."

The following description of the specific object, however, then again recalls Freud's shadow: This hostile and envious object becomes a "Super-Ego": "'Somewhere' there is present a 'super-ego' that is cruel, denuded of all the characteristics usually associated with the super-ego, and, finally, of 'existence' itself. It therefore has the characteristics of 'non-existence'..." (Bion, 1970, 21)

It is a super-ego that has hardly any of the characteristics of the super-ego as understood in psycho-analysis: it is "super" ego. It is an envious assertion of moral superiority without any morals... The process of denudation continues till – ♂ – ♀ represent hardly more than an empty superiority-inferiority that in turn degenerates to nullity.

(Bion, 1962, 97; also 1965, 64)

While Bion continues to try to describe the super-ego as a kind of inner object, de facto it is a matter of "to be or not to be", an attempt to "intuit" "non-existence", the dark throbbing of the ulterior, unthinkable extinction, to hear "the voice of breakdown" (Eshel, 2016) or "a voice from the crypt" (Grotstein, 2010, cited in Eshel, 2016, 85).

At the same time, however, Bion made the important discovery of the failure of projective identification: Projective identification can fail since it requires the recognition of objects. The projection of personality aspects is precluded "because there is no conception of containers into which the projection could take place" (Bion, 1970, 12). But here, too, Bion refers back to Kleinian models of projection: Thus, explosive projection follows – in a space that is so vast that "the patient's capacity for emotion is felt to be lost because emotion itself is felt to drain away and be lost in the immensity" (12). "The mental realization of space is therefore felt as an immensity so great that it cannot be represented even by astronomical space because it cannot be represented at all" (12).

But what if not only projective identification fails, but projection (as evacuation) fails altogether? If the disruption occurs at a time when time and space, inside and outside, self and object, are not yet securely given? How is something to be expelled that is not represented, indeed that is "non-existent"? Is explosive infinite space to be distinguished from the implosive, infinitely condensed point? This perspective is closer to clinical empiricism: Many patients feel that the state of non-existence cannot be expelled, but is sometimes dark, sometimes silent, sometimes throbbing omnipresent.

This is precisely the direction of investigation taken by Winnicott, whose concept of breakdown is probably clinically closest to the state of non-existence:

> ... the breakdown has already happened, near the beginning of the individual's life. The patient needs to "remember" this but it is not possible to remember something that has not yet happened, and this thing of the past has not happened yet because the patient was not there for it to happen to. The only way to "remember" in this case is for the patient to experience this past thing for the first time in the present, that is to say, in the transference. This past and future thing then becomes a matter of the here and now, and becomes experienced by the patient for the first time.
>
> (Winnicott, 1974, 105)

This breakdown has occurred in the time of absolute dependence, ego and non-ego are not yet (safely) separated. The breakdown is "hidden away in the unconscious" (104), but this unconscious is not the repressed unconscious or that of the neurophysiological functioning, or the unconscious of Jung. Such actual-traumatic encapsulations thus do not show the classical traumatic features that visualisations or impressions leave behind: "To understand this it is necessary to think not of trauma but of nothing happening when something might profitably have happened" (106). Psychotic phenomena may therefore represent defences against breakdowns that disguise the actual abyss: "It is wrong to think of psychotic illness as a breakdown, it is a defence organisation relative to primitive agony..." (104).

Ultimately, it is about a breakdown of going on being. What does that mean? I think of it this way: The continuity of being is interrupted, being then continues without it being possible to connect to the previous state. There remains a void that cannot be filled, but also cannot be psychically grasped, certainly not represented – not even afterwards. The body has lived on, the "psyche" has suffered death. An annihilation that has occurred as "nothing" or "void."

Winnicott works with a different concept of object than Freud and Bion and therefore sees failure of the facilitating environment at work. (But it is noticeable that he is relatively economical by his standards with this causal attribution in this work.) But this failure cannot explain the intrapsychic and interpsychic dynamics.

1.3   Autistic and autistoid states

The observations of Bion, Winnicott and Meltzer then led to a series of further investigations. One of the psychoanalytic directions that studied nameless states in the broad sense had its starting point in the study of early childhood autism.

Along with Mahler, Bettelheim and others, Tustin's work (1972, 1980, 1981, 1984, 1986, 1988) with children on the autistic spectrum made clear that "concepts such as encapsulation, imitative fusion, autistic objects and autistic shapes, as defences against the 'black hole' of nonrelationship, are ... descriptive of the autistic child's reactions" (1988, 39).

The traumatic, too early separation from the mother is felt as a loss of the rudimentary self and object (breast), which, sensed physically-concretely, leaves a hole at the mouth and breast: "a traumatic awareness of separateness occurred in the state of being an 'emergent self', and before 'the core of the self' had developed" (Tustin, 1986, 23). Autistic defences develop which "divert attention away from this mother, who is spurned in favour of self-generated sensations which are always available and predictable, and so do not bring shocks" (Tustin, 1986, 27). (In these self-generated states, psychic objects are indistinguishable from things like furniture. Tustin refers here to M. Klein's early observations in Dick (Klein, 1930).) "The encapsulating reactions support and protect the damaged part and shut out the fear of being killed but, metaphorically speaking, their psychic functioning is frozen and immobilized" (Tustin, 1986, 25). In a desperate search, the dangers of dissolution are resisted by formations which centre the sensations (a lamp, a voice, a smell or others) and can thus, at least momentarily, be experienced "as holding the parts of the personality together" (Bick, 1968, 484).

The discovery that there are also autistic barriers and phenomena in neurotic patients (see Bick, Meltzer, Tustin, S. Klein) then made problems in treatments more understandable. Autistic and autistoid features could be identified in almost all personalities; therefore the diagnosis also changed to autistic spectrum disorders. The sensitisation for such parts made it clear that there can also be autistic and autistoid parts in "normal" or "neurotic" personalities, which can have a malignant effect in the relationship and in psychic life. If they are not recognised or are treated in the wrong way technically, e.g. if they are interpreted symbolically or in the transference, they cannot be worked on and can lead to stagnation and dead ends.

In further work it became more and more irrefutable that such states are not (sufficiently) psychicised and have fallen out of the objectal dynamic: Projective identification fails, hope for containment is lost, raw sensual elements and unrealised preconceptions lead to strangeness in the world. These autistic and autistoid states can manifest themselves in a variety of symptoms:

S. Klein (1980) described psychosomatic states as autistic encapsulation. As early as 1984, David Rosenfeld was already making sophisticated reflections on "autistoid" hypochondria and examined, among other things, drug addiction under this focus (2006). Innes-Smith (1987) describes patients with "pockets of autistic functioning." Gomberoff, Noemi and Gomberoff (1990) discuss autistic objects in transference and countertransference, focusing among other things on the connection between language and communication. Mitrani discusses several case studies, including fibromyalgia as a chronic use of auto-sensory protective factors and presents different transient symptoms to be noted as autistoid (2009).

Cohen and Jay (1996) discuss case studies with encapsulated and "entangled" borderline patients. Klüwer (1997, 2006), among others, shows the connection to the as-ob (as-if) syndrome. Furthermore, there are numerous other contributions to specific pathologies such as K. Barrows (1999) on eating disorders or Asseyer (2002) on obsessive-compulsive disorder or Nissen as well as Schellekes on hypochondria (Nissen, 2000, 2015a, 2018; Schellekes, 2017) and Nissen on perversion

(2009). In 2014, I tried to show that the identification of autistoid features can be diagnostically and indicatively important in the preliminary examination (initial interview). In further publications, De Cesarei (2005) describes an autistic core in bipolarity to a developed narcissism and Fix Korbivcher proposes the assumption of an autistic transformation (2005, 2014). Strauss (2006) presents an analysis of an adult male who was diagnosed with Asperger's symptoms and discusses treatment considerations ("forced interpretations") in 2014. Beland (2012) describes autistoid thought disorders in a severe super-ego pathology. Schneider (2006) outlines a borderline disorder with severe psychotic phases in which a broad core area of psychological and external being is characterised by autistic phenomena. (For an overview, see e.g. Nissen, 2006, 2008; Barrows, 2008; Mitrani & Mitrani, 2015; Levine & Power, 2017; Rhode, 2018).

More and more the concept of the autistic object was defined by the function, so that even stories (Barrows, 2001), for instance, or the voice, are seen as autistic objects (e.g. Rhode, 1997). The patients console themselves in a two-dimensional world of sensations, which are so refined that they are then the subject of a cognitive processing which frequently leads to an impressive keenness and brilliance of observation, description and intellect, yet are no longer transformed into a psychic state and thus are not available to the mental system, perpetuating the unintegrated state and encouraging the singularisation of the sensory apparatus. Ogden (1989, 1992), conceptualises, together with the paranoid-schizoid and depressive, an autistic-contiguous position, which he does not see as a system that is closed to the object world but as a modus in which object relations are experienced in the form of sensory surfaces.

This different experience of self, object, relationship and world also shows up clinically-atmospherically in the treatments: Almost all the authors speak of the absence of an unconscious flow and emotional exchange in autistoid patients, of frequently unnoticed "static situations" (Fix Korbivcher, 2005) and non-understanding, registering the failure of projective identification; there is also talk of standstill, shallowness (Meltzer, 1975b, 235), an emotional void and levelling out; Innes-Smith (1987) describes patients with "pockets of autistic functioning" (405). In the treatment, the absence of normal resonance is shown, feelings of "non-being" (de Cesarei, 2005), the inability to mentalise communications as emotional experiences (Strauss, 2006), the absence of involvements (cf. Klüwer, 2006) develop, but also partial fusions of patient and analyst, who in this way, frequently unnoticed by the analyst, establish a common "autistic object." Gomberoff et al. say:

> The patient may establish the autistic object by taking aspects of the setting or from the analyst, the latter not being aware of what is going on. In other cases, the patient acts, urging the analyst to answer, which becomes a repeating situation.
>
> (Gomberoff et al., 1990, 253)

What is crucial is that the traumas that occur here encounter an immature self, more precisely an infant that has not yet been able to develop a self-core and a (safe) self-object differentiation. The "not-me" was not separated from the "me," so no me was there for it to happen to (see Winnicott).[2] These states are therefore not *psychically* presented.

These approaches, in contrast to e.g. theory of mind research (e.g. Frith, 1991; Baron-Cohon, 2000), examine the consequences of early traumatic disorders object-theoretically, i.e. the disorder is conceived as one that occurred in the earliest object relationship. The economic point of view has not been central for a long time, unlike psychoanalytic trauma theory, which examines both psycho-economic and object relations approaches. These theories conceptualise trauma as a breach of the "protective shield" (Freud, 1920g, 27) of the psychic space with the release of overpowering, destructive fear, so that a state of extreme agitation, of objectlessness and helplessness occurs, leaving behind an unintegrated "space." As a consequence, not only does symbolisation break down, but also the giving of meaning and psychic element formation. The sense of time changes, too, by "freezing up." Roussillon also speaks of the psychic being "petrified" (Roussillon, 2021, 204) or "frozen up" (Roussillon, 2021, 205) in traumatic disorders.

Traumas can be based on singular events, be the result of long-term stress (Kris, 1956) or build up cumulatively (Khan, 1963) (for an overview, see Bohleber, 2002).

However, these trauma-theoretical considerations mostly assume a developed self that is capable of object relations. Early traumatisation, as described in the autistic spectrum, is not about a breakdown of an existing object relationship, but about a non-realisation of objectal expectations and thus about a breakdown of the earliest self-experience. Therefore, the classic characteristics of trauma such as intrusion, flash-back, etc., are usually non-existent. It has more the characteristics of the void, of nothingness, of non-existence.

1.4   "White states" in French psychoanalysis

In France, another current emerged (see Aisenstein, 2006) that examined deficiencies in psychic representation. This Parisian psychosomatic school described dynamics in which a peculiar "flattening" and tendency towards the concrete was evident, with an apparent inability to fantasise and freely associate. These states were referred to, among other things, by the terms "relation blanche" and operative thinking ("pensée opératoire"): "It is a conscious thinking which (1) seems to have no internal relation with an accessible phantasy activity; which (2) reproduces the action like an image, sometimes preceding it or – in a limited period of time – following it" (Marty et al., 1978 (1963), 974; transl. BN). "But the peculiarity of this thinking consists above all in not signifying (signifier) the action – giving it a meaning – but merely duplicating it: the word merely repeats what the hand does at work" (Marty et al., 1978, 977; transl. BN).

Without the therapist's activities, the conversations threaten to die out:

> The sick person often shows no interest in us. He simply waits for the questions, which he answers almost mechanically, without any attempt to associate. Since he makes no effort at all and the conversation does not proceed spontaneously, an "energetic contribution" must be made several times, questions and encouragement must be used to prevent the conversation from petering out.
>
> (de M'Uzan, 1977, 319; transl. BN)

1.4.1   Green's "clinic of the negative"

The "series" of blankness ("white series") was then continued by Green: negative hallucination, blank psychosis and blank mourning. "Winnicott's intuitive insights into negative processes" were for Green "the basis for his conception and elaboration of the negative" (2009, 135; transl. BN).[3] Green redefines the relationship between life instinct and death instinct with his construction of a positive and a negative primary narcissism (see also 1975). The life instinct seeks attachment and objectalisation functions, the death instinct detachment and disobjectalisation functions (2001): The "temptation of nothingness is … the real meaning of the death drive" (2001, 532; transl. BN). It is the tendency of "the ego to undo its unity and to proceed towards nought. This is clinically manifest by the feeling of emptiness" (Green, 2005, 167). In this view, the death drive, in deviation from Freud in my opinion, acquires a structuring presence and immediate effectiveness, so that the dynamics of the death drive become investigable like those of the life drives.

Unlike "red anxiety" as a result of castration anxiety/castration associated with a bloody deed, the "clinic of the negative" or the "clinic of emptiness" is characterised by a

> massive decathexis, both radical and temporary, which leaves traces in the unconscious in the form of "psychical holes". These will be filled in by recathexes, which are the expression of destructiveness which has thus been freed by the weakening of libidinal erotic cathexis.
>
> (Green, 2005, 146)

Green arrives at the complex of the "dead mother" via this, where a living, cathected object has fallen into a severe depression, brutally transformed "into a distant figure, toneless, practically inanimate" (Green, 2005, 142): "Thus, the dead mother, contrary to what one might think, is a mother who remains alive but who is, so to speak, psychically dead in the eyes of the young child in her care" (142). Green combines findings from the "white line" with his clinical observations and concludes that the following has happened:

> The object has been encapsulated and its trace has been lost through decathexis; primary identification with the dead mother took place, transforming positive

identification into negative identification, i.e. identification with the hole left by the decathexis (and not identification with the object), and to this emptiness, which is filled in and suddenly manifests itself through an affective hallucination of the dead mother, as soon as a new object is periodically chosen to occupy this space.

(Green, 2005, 155)

Loss of meaning is inextricably linked to this dynamic.

Accompanying this dynamic are secondary manifestations: black hatred directed at the father (152); autoerotic excitations on the level of pure sensual pleasure, organ pleasure (152); a hunt in quest of an unintrojectable object (153).

As I understand Green, a child who has objectally cathected the mother and already has a somewhat developed self has had to experience his mother falling into a severe depression. A positively cathected object and a satisfied relationship disintegrate into a negative emptiness and a stifled relationship. The small child thus experiences two very different states, resulting in a pressure of psychic operations to cope with the traumatic situation – which does not succeed. The withdrawal of cathexis led to a primary identification with the dead object which, via negative identification, led to an identification with the void.

The undoubtedly traumatic experience of the disintegration of a vital mother into a dead one also means a dying off of parts of the self. Is primary identification still possible for such a weakened self? Is it even possible in the traumatic to identify with a dead object? Green breaks down the notion of primary identification to the notion of mimicry (151), i.e. a mechanism that is not psychic but an adhesive adaptation (see Meltzer: adhesive identification 1975c; Mitrani: adhesive equation, 2012). The traumatic takes such forms that it is experienced as a hole, later emptiness. How can there still be identification in such states, which may approach Winnicott's breakdown in terms of traumatic severity? In my opinion, the secondary phenomena mentioned above are also more reminiscent of the perverse excitations that so often surround the traumatic core: excited attempts to expel the traumatic, resulting in rejection of an object; excitations acted perversely on the body, never relaxing; the desperate attempts to penetrate to the traumatic core, never succeeding. Green's answer might be that there was a positive, living cathexis before the depressive death, so the child remains dynamically attached to the mother in repetitions.

But the question remains how to think about the fundamental structural-dynamic and clinical differences between traumatic events that at one time acted before the establishment of a core self, and at another time encounter a developed self and an object relationship.

What these very different approaches have in common is that they start from a traumatic core that is not psychically presented, let alone represented (for the distinction "to present" – "darstellen" – "to represent" – "vorstellen," see Kahn, 2013), that persists actual, seems to resist all changes and corresponds with the abandonment of objectal hope, not infrequently falling out of the communication from unconscious to unconscious.

But Green goes further, not stopping at this clinical-descriptive analysis. He interprets Freudian psychology from the second topic and develops a model that has gained strong influence on the psychoanalytic movement that studies "unrepresented states." As this model is of utmost importance, I quote Green at length, who summarises his reflections in a condensed form in his work "On Construction in Freud's Work":

> It will be worthwhile to throw more light on the circumstances in which we resort to interpretation and construction. It seems to me that the recourse to construction is not indispensable in cases of neurotic patients, for their psychic functions are intact and they produce spontaneous constructions more or less by themselves. On the other hand, when we are dealing with patients who can only be understood in terms of the second topography, that is, where the representative agencies are more or less out of play, construction becomes indispensable. In the first case, construction remains silent in the analyst, or at least is used to a limited extent. On the contrary, in the second case, the analytic work makes recourse to construction almost obligatory.
>
> In other words the relations between the agencies Cs-Pcs-Ucs permit this form of psychoanalytic creativity, grounded in the transference, although the role of resistance must not be neglected. The raison d'être for this situation is that the functions of representation, which are an integral part of the unconscious structures, are absent from the theorizations on the id, as Freud suggests. Here the instinctual impulses now play the role formerly attributed to unconscious representations. We must not forget that since the Ego and the Id (Freud, 1923), Freud has dethroned the unconscious from the place that he had hitherto attributed to it. The unconscious pursues its activities but is now attached to the unconscious structures of the ego, remaining out of reach of the id, which, for Freud, is rooted in the somatic. Analytic work will endeavour to transform the expressions of the instinctual impulses into unconscious representations to facilitate the transformation of thing-presentations into word-presentations, a transition that is illustrated by verbalization. When this transition cannot be accomplished, it is because it is hampered by archaic anxieties.
>
> Historical truth is subjective truth inasmuch as it is connected with what appeared to be real and true at a certain moment in the subject's history. At this time, only the subjective object exists for the psyche which does not as yet have the possibility of cathecting the objectively perceived object, which is felt to be independent of the subject and placed outside him (Winnicott).
>
> This throws light on the modern clinical experience of non-neurotic structures which present various forms of repetition-compulsion: acting out, somatizations, hallucinatory episodes, states of depersonalization, negative therapeutic reactions, etc.
>
> (Green, 2012, 1241f)

Green's emphasis on construction in "degrading" interpretation is carried out by Freud himself in his work (1937d). More importantly, however, in the "second topography the representative agencies are ... out of play" and "the functions of representation, which are an integral part of the unconscious structures, are absent from the theorizations on the id." These functions are now attributed to the ego – "remaining out of reach of the id, which, for Freud, is rooted in the somatic." The id becomes the reservoir of the drives or drive energies. A dethronement of the unconscious, indeed. (Laplanche and Pontalis, 1972, see it the other way round: the id as a kind of castrated system Ucs.) "Analytic work will endeavour to transform the expressions of the instinctual impulses into unconscious representations." If this transition is hindered, archaic anxieties are to be discerned. Historical truth is subjective truth and is connected with the subjective object. Green then mentions some clinical phenomena that can be better understood (e.g. acting out, somatisations, hallucinations, negative therapeutic reactions, etc.). There are still some side notes to be marked, which also had a great impact: The first topography has proven effective for neurotic patients, for their psychic functions are intact. Furthermore, Green seems to establish a connection between the agencies Cs-Pcs-Ucs and psychoanalytic creativity, grounded in the transference, "although the role of resistance must not be neglected." Can we conclude from this that in "unrepresented states" transference plays no or a subordinate role? To clarify, nameless (unrepresented) states are not objectal, but does it follow from this that transference plays no role?

Are Green's reflections now an interpretation of Freudian psychology from the perspective of the second topography[4] or is it not rather a new draft of a Greenian metapsychology?

Freud describes the id as

the dark, inaccessible part of our personality; what little we know of it we have learnt from our study of the dream-work and of the construction of neurotic symptoms, and most of that is of a negative character and can be described only as a contrast to the ego. We approach the id with analogies: we call it a chaos, a cauldron full of seething excitations. We picture it as being open at its end to somatic influences, and *as there taking up into itself instinctual needs which find their psychical expression in it*, but we cannot say in what substratum. It is filled with energy reaching it from the instincts, but it has no organization, produces no collective will, but only a striving to bring about the satisfaction of the instinctual needs subject to the observance of the pleasure principle.

(Freud, 1933a, 73; italics BN)

However, he then goes on to list again the characteristics he has already elaborated in the work "The Unconscious," e.g. invalidity of the logical laws of thought, no negation, timelessness, etc. The repressed is a part of the id:

But the repressed merges into the id as well, and is merely a part of it. The repressed is only cut off sharply from the ego by the resistances of repression; it can communicate with the ego through the id.

(1923b, 24)

The id is the reservoir of the drives that find their psychical expression in it, i.e. the drives are psychically represented in the id.[5] It also contains the repressed and is open to the ego. Central features of the Ucs system have thus been preserved. Even though the id is a cauldron full of seething excitations, the laws of the unconscious still apply (primary process, pleasure principle, symmetrical logics, etc.). For Green, however, the pathological phenomena listed as various forms of repetition compulsion seem to be expressions of somatic, thus unrepresented instinctual impulses. But what are the conditions for the impulse not finding its psychical expression?

With Green, it could be argued that a subject as a differentiated self has had positive object relation experiences, i.e. the drive has found its object and is psychically represented. If this object relational possibility breaks down, the drive can no longer find psychical expression and remains an instinctual impulse, trapped in ruminant repetition compulsion. Green's theory would then be limited to a phenomenal area in which a developed self capable of object relations encounters traumatic experiences of loss. However, the concept of trauma here corresponds neither to the traumatic experience before the constitution of a core self nor to that of trauma theory in the narrower sense.

1.4.2   Regredience

A clinical-theoretical application of the concept of the negative has been presented by S. Botella (2005), C. & S. Botella (2005, 2013) and C. Botella (2014).

They focus on "the problematic of a core of mental states without representation…" (2013, 95). They transpose Freud's dream theory, based in the first topical model, to the structural model and develop a theory of regredience to deal with these states.

Such state exists as

> a quantity of energy that has remained like a foreign body, without form or shape, without representation or memory, and even less meaning, and which can only be discharged through action or the hallucinatory activity of dreams by making use of any context whatsoever. Its content is more or less a matter of indifference; the only thing that counts is the repetition of the affect irrespective of the content used to convey it.
>
> (Botella, 2014, 915)

In their opinion, Freud abandoned the potentialities present in the metapsychology of "interpretation of dreams" (1900a) in favour of a "theory of neurosis" (2013, 97) in which an attempt is made to make repressed memories conscious with the help of the techniques of transference and transference neurosis that have become central (see Green above). Memories are understood here as repressed factual realities. C. Botella puts it very pointedly: Freud

> … then developed the conception of a sort of "memory funnel" governing the treatment in which the analyst is only interested in what flows from it, that

is to say the recollection of repressed infantile experience. The analyst should hear nothing else. Infantile amnesia was redefined in the sense of the theory of repression as the amnesia of memory-traces, historical "remnants" of a past registered as memory.

(2014, 917)

In this attitude, it is not possible to gain access to the contents of "memory without recollection." Much like Green, C. Botella postulates: "the theory of neurosis is only a part of Freudian thought, only a sector of psychic life; it no longer represents the whole of psychic life" (2014, 913).

According to C. & S. Botella, Freud only returned to the potentialities of dream interpretation in the wake of the works of 1920 & 1923, when in 1933a he corrected the wish fulfilment of the dream and spoke of the "attempt at the fulfilment of a wish" (1933a, 29). They then see the second fundamental change in the work "constructions in analysis." This means that the search for remembered, repressed facts is no longer central, but that mechanisms of the dream can be used to discover unrepresented states. For this, they refer to the term "regredient" which, in their opinion, should be defined differently from regression [6] Freud's observation is used: "We call it 'regression' when in a dream an idea is turned back into the sensory image from which it was originally derived" (1900a, 543; in German: regression = Regression; idea = Vorstellung). Botella and Botella define regredience as follows:

"Regredience" is a psychic state that includes quality and movement in an evolving process; it offers a potential for transformation, a permanent psychic capacity for transforming in an endohallucinatory manner any quantity of excitation, verbal, motor, or emotional. The dream is its most accomplished manifestation.

(In Botella, 2014, 919)

This capacity of the dream can be used technically if it is possible to get into an attitude of recasting the material of the session into sensory images (Freud, 1900a, 547). The presentability (figurability) of the dream is used (see Freud, Chapter VI, Part C; see also Kahn, 2013, 125f: "figurability or presentability?"). With an attitude that is open to regredient processes, unrepresented states can be grasped and used for constructions in the sense of Freud that gain the rank of conviction, i.e. are completely equivalent to memory.

S. Botella (2005; see also Kittler, 2022, who discusses this position very knowledgeably) provides a theoretical model: No dream thoughts can be formed because the arousals are like an imprint without imagination, memory without recollection. The analyst has to do the dream-work for the patient: "The regredient hallucinatory movement follows a sensory trace and in the 'flash' grabs a figure that charges itself with meaning as it becomes conscious..." (Kittler, 2022, 919; transl. BN). Since the Botellas, like Green, conceive of the id only as a cauldron full of seething excitations, which is filled up with energy from the drives (Freud, 1933a, 80), conscious and unconscious are not understood as systems, but as processual activities.

Then the question becomes compelling as to how the transformation into the psychic can succeed. Hallucinatory wish fulfilment must therefore have a preliminary process – the work of figurability. S. Botella (2005, 717ff) refers to Peirce and his theory of categories: firstness, secondness, thirdness: "A sensation connects with a thought, a judgement through the mediation of a force (secondness), which itself is thoughtless, unimaginative, groundless, without sense or reason, and which only experiences itself through an obstacle, an object" (Kittler, 2022, 923f; transl. BN). Without knowing it, Oedipus kills his father, who stands in his way, with impulsive violence. It is only afterwards ("nachträglich") that he is able to grasp the event psychologically.[7]

At first, according to the Botellas, there are only sensual and mnestic impressions that do not connect to memory images – memory without recollection. This is where the work of figurability comes in, in which the analyst hallucinatively combines and psychicises sensual and mnestic impressions for the patient, so that the patient can finally "dream."

But are the sensual and mnestic impressions not based on realised experiences, i.e. on qualified preconceptions/conceptions? Is there then memory without recollection? Doesn't the regredient figurability presuppose imagination (Vorstellungen) and sensual perception? Does the theory of figurability and regredience solve the basic problem of psychisation, for which Bion tried to offer a solution with his idea of an α-structured pre-conception?

These approaches of French psychoanalysis start from the negative (or Botella from the negative of trauma), i.e. from states that have no meaning, are not processed as unconscious fantasies. The negative primary narcissism (death drive) stands in difference to a fulfilled positive primary narcissism (life instincts); both drives are localised in the id. With the broad version of the death drive, which is conceived as present, active and virulent, and the redefinition of the id, emptiness, negative of trauma, etc., can be understood as unrepresented states, as psychic reality beyond the repressed.

1.5   Unrepresented states

More recently, the approaches of Green and C. & S. Botella have been linked with work by Bion and examined under the focus of "unrepresented states and the construction of meaning" (the book title of Levine, Reed and Scarfone (ed.), 2013).

Defining the negative positively is not easy. The concepts of the unrepresented are based on Green, but in my opinion they define these states more broadly. Reed (2013), for example, speaks of "an empty mirror," Levine of "the colourless canvas." For Levine

the clinical manifestations of the failure or weakening of representation include the all-too-familiar range of impulsive, eruptive, destructive, and self-destructive feelings and actions with which we, and our patients, are so often confronted. This is the provenance of affect storms, impulsive actions, blind and peremptory discharge phenomena, extreme states of psychic deadness and stasis, somatic breakdowns, rigid pathological organizations, severe negative therapeutic reactions, perversions, addictions, destructive unconscious guilt, and so on.

(Levine, 2013, 53)

Levine locates "unrepresented states" in the "unstructured unconscious" (Levine, 2013, 43; 2022, 39; 2023): "In addition to a repressed unconscious, we may now speak of an *unstructured unconscious* that consists of forces, unqualified sensations and turbulences that are unrepresented or unrepresentable" (Levine, 2023). In the unstructured unconscious, the not yet psychically represented exists and is separated from the represented by a β-screen. With reference to Chapter 10 of Bion's *Learning through Experience* (1962), the β-screen allows the psyche to relieve itself of stimulus increases. Levine sees unrepresented dynamics at work here – he explicitly corrects Bion at this point – not psychotic ones. This kind of elimination leads to emotional entanglements "by unconscious emotional induction" (Levine, 2023), which can then be used by a trained intuition.

But is there conscious and unconscious in systemic terms in the failure of α-function and the establishment of a β-screen? Bion speaks of "an inability to dream through lack of alpha-elements and therefore an inability to sleep or wake, to be either conscious or unconscious" (1962, 21) and the resulting states in which, for example, the analyst is conscious but incapable of the functions of consciousness and the patient is unconscious incapable of the functions of unconsciousness (Bion, 1962, 21). I.e. if the α-function collapses or is not established, the functions of consciousness and unconsciousness break down: "It is unsuited to the establishment of conscious and unconscious, and therefore conducive to defective or anomalous developments of a capacity for memory and repression" (1962, 22).

Lombardi (2016; see also concise summary in Zeitzschel, 2017), following Matte Blanco, also speaks of an "unrepressed unconscious" or "structural unconscious." The application of symmetrical logic leads to infinite sets. Therefore the "unconscious requires what Matte Blanco calls a 'translation function', or better still, 'unfolding', in order to transform it into something 'thinkable'" (Lombardi, 2009a, 537). Symmetrical logic is necessary for the development of thinking, but according to Lombardi it must also be anchored in the thinkable:

The symmetric-asymmetric oscillation is, for Matte Blanco, constantly involved in mental functioning. Phenomena of sensory saturation, linked to emotional intensity, lead the mind to a continuous slide towards infinitization of emotions, to the point of jeopardizing the work of the unfolding function. This function is adept at transforming phenomena which are largely "symmetric" into phenomena that are largely "asymmetric".

(Lombardi, 2009a, 541)

If this function fails, impressions and sensations can become extremely intense, unthinkable and disintegrating. Therefore, for Lombardi, the body occupies a central position. With Ferrari (2004), Lombardi distinguishes a horizontal axis of relation between analyst and analysand from a vertical body-soul axis in the analysand, which can be decoded through reverie and perception of one's own body sensations.[8] With his precise investigations of the vertical axis (vertical relation), Lombardi (2009b) opens up important perspectives on nameless states.

Bergstein, not unlike Levine and Lombardi, assumes an "unrepressed unconscious" (e.g. 2014, 2018, 2020), which he defines as follows:

> Repressed unconscious experiences may be represented; hence they can appear in dreams, slips of the tongue, symptoms and so on and can be brought into consciousness by interpretation. However when we speak of unrepressed unconscious, we refer to impressions that are without representation and so do not require specific mental activity to keep them from consciousness. Even so, their presence is betrayed by the emergence of baffling and disturbing behaviours, as well as pre-representational experiential elements, uncanny sensations stirred up, not yet formed into any coherent image, unmentalized and irrepresentable. These may include sensory impressions, stereotyped actions, physiological reactions, posture, intonations and rhythms of speech, and isolated fragmented images or affects. These often hang loosely together and do not usually lead to a well-formed understanding in the analyst's mind that can be usefully fed back as an interpretation....
>
> (2014, 852)

Bergstein also suspects encapsulations here (2020, 866).

Bergstein also introduces Bion's term "inaccessible part of the personality":

> Bion (1977c) describes an unconscious mental state that has never been anything else, has never been conscious. He suggests that in addition to unconscious and conscious states of mind there may be another state of mind, one that might provisionally be called an inaccessible state of mind. Bion tries to address this inaccessible part that has remained as a meaningless frenzy in the psyche. He thus tries to approach "a mental life unmapped by theories elaborated for the understanding of neurosis" (Bion 1962, p. 37).
>
> (2018, 202)

Bergstein, however, summarily sets this inaccessible state congruent with his concept of the unrepressed unconscious, which hardly seems possible to me, since Bion explicitly defines it as not conscious and not unconscious.

Bergstein and Levine thus locate the nameless in the non-repressed unconscious. But as explained, the unconscious is the real psychic, and Freud goes further: It is subject to laws (primary process; pleasure, unpleasure principle; symmetrical logic), is "alive and capable of development and maintains a number of other relations with the Pcs. ... [and] ... is continued into what are known as derivatives, that it is accessible to the impressions of life..." (1915e, 190; also Matte-Blanco, 1998).

How are the unrepresented states to be thought of in this "wider unconscious"? Are they excluded from the dynamics or yet – as with Green – involved even if they become unrepresentable?

The answer could be found in the fact that Green, but increasingly Levine, Bergstein and others identify a shift in Freud's theoretical and technical focus, a shift from a "theory centered on psychic *contents* (…) to a theory about *process* and the movements needed to tame the unstructured, not yet represented aspects of *the drive* – that is, emotion, impulse and somatic discharge – within the psychic apparatus" (Levine, 2023). I.e. the focus shifts from the content to the processes in the unrepressed unconscious. Bergstein (2022) refers here to Bion's theory of observation in which *the processes* are observed by which an emotional experience is transformed and represented. Bion seems to me to be referring to Winnicott in these processes (see also Aguayo, 2018). Winnicott writes: "… the patient must go on looking for the past detail which is not yet experienced. This search takes the form of a looking for this detail in the future" (Winnicott, 1974, 105). Bion states:

Similarly, the patient may express a fear of the future which has many of the characteristies of a past which one thinks he could not possibly remember, nor can he remember the future because it has not yet happened. These things, so faintly expressed, may in truth be very powerful. I can imagine that there may be ideas which cannot be more powerfully expressed because they are buried in the future which has not happened, or buried in the past which is forgotten, and which can hardly be said to belong to what we call "thought."

(Bion, 1975, 38–39)

Bion elaborates: "The past what is known, interpretations which are given and so on, those are very rapidly of no importance; *the present and the future which hasn't happened yet, **that** is important*" (Bion, quoted after Bergstein, 2022). On this basis, Bergstein now comes to the following conclusion:

Bion is concerned with the *observation of the evolution*, or the transformation of the emotional experience, evolving into the future, in the immediacy of the here and now of the session, and it is that which he will want to interpret and help the patient get in touch with. Only that evolving reality is experience-near, available to both patient and analyst. Hence it can be apprehended and not only talked *about*.

(2022)

In other words, the processes of the unrepressed unconscious can only be intuited in the here and now, but they always evolve into the future.

For me, the question remains whether the unconscious is not timeless, as Freud postulates it to be.[9] Then what seems to come from the future can be a past event, as described by Winnicott.

In this conception of process, emphasis is placed on the permanent changes in the psychic (see also Bion, 1975). This in fact introduces a new concept of content. The psychic entity "deed," as Freud calls it (1926e; also Nissen, 2019), is no longer central; the constructivist element dominates.

But it seems to me that the definition of the subject area is not really possible yet, even the "location" remains vague: Are such states or processes non-psychicised, i.e. neither conscious nor unconscious complexes, and thus not part of the unrepressed unconscious? Or are they psychic complexes in a wider unconscious that have no meaning yet? I think these questions cannot be decided at the moment.

For me, the nameless has the characteristics of the non-psychicised, the objectless and the actual. The nameless is neither conscious nor unconscious and, since the objectal hope is dispersed, hardly leads into emotional entanglements. These states, and clinical empiricism shows this, are hidden away or encapsulated.

Elsewhere (Nissen, 2023) I have asked whether the nameless lies beyond the unconscious. But can nameless states be completely excluded from psychic intercourse? They are, after all, represented (though not psychically), so must at some point show themselves temporarily or locally in the psychoanalytic process. How can this relationship, which probably only appears binary in the strict theoretical decomposition, be determined? It would also be conceivable that they lie as non-psychic in the middle of the psychic, but do not belong to the psychic and are excluded from psychic processes. This perspective would better explain the recognition of nameless states. For, as with somatic encapsulations, psychic processes must organise themselves around the nameless. The nameless states are discoverable, changeable, and must retain – in whatever form – something of the events that have not been experienced.

Perhaps an appropriate image would be that of an analogue photograph. The (traumatic) event would then be the exposure of the film, in photographic language: a latent picture. This latent picture exists, but has yet to become; for without chemical treatment it cannot appear. With chemical development, it can become a negative, and then finally become a photograph, a positive. The event (early childhood trauma) is experienced in the transference (negative picture) in order to then become a thought, conceivable (developed picture) in the further process.

Notes

1 Angeloch makes an exciting attempt to connect Bion's theory and writings with the biographical background, which is helpful for understanding Bion's work:

All his life, Wilfred Bion attempted to devise a narrative form for an account of the traumatic experiences he went through as a tank commander in the First World War. The body of his autobiographical works, which consists of texts written in different stages of his life and remain fragmentary, documents his desperate efforts to wrest a biography of his own from the most appalling tendencies of world history. As a whole, it testifies for and is the result of a lifelong attempt to understand something incomprehensible, to express something unspeakable, to restore something destroyed.... Taken together, these sequences impressively show the painful work of gradually dissolving or at least coming to terms with the psychological catastrophe of a paralyzing trauma, the causes of which reach far beyond the individual and the private.

(Angeloch, 2021, 7–8)

2 Bush des Ahumada & Ahumada have impressively shown in their clinical examples what a turning point the differentiation I-You means in the work with children from the autistic spectrum (e.g. 2009, 2017).
3 It is interesting that Freud already speaks of the negative in 1917: "I may add by way of supplement that any attempt to explain hallucination would have to start out from negative rather than positive hallucination" (1917d, 232).
4 There are many reasons for the development of the second topography, e.g. the pressure from clinical observation that defence and resistance are unconscious, in which another instance (superego) is relevant and cannot be grasped with the previous systems Ucs, Pcs and Cs. Another reason, in my opinion, is that the system (sic!) Cs could not really be conceptualised. Still in the "Outline," Freud writes that consciousness is "fact without parallel, which defies all explanation or description" (1940a, 157); see also Freud's speculation that "*consciousness arises instead of a memory-trace*" (1920g, 25; also 1925a).
5 The definition of drive and psychic representation is not clear in Freud's work (see e.g. 1905d, 1911c, 1915c, 1915e, 1920g, 1923b, 1933a): At times there seems to be no distinction between drive and psychic representation; at other times there is a clear separation between the idea that represents it and the drive. For example, Strachey writes in a footnote (1933a): "Freud is here regarding instincts as something physical, of which mental processes are the representatives" (footnote 2 of Strachey, in Freud 1933a, 73).
6 I don't see the differences so clearly. Freud does not use the terms distinctly.
7 I cannot follow S. Botella's interpretation of the Oedipus tragedy. According to S. Botella, Oedipus kills his father "in self-defence" and in the impossibility of recognising his father, of knowing him, even of seeing him (2005, 724). I assume that father (Laius) and son (Oedipus) unconsciously knew who they had before them.
8 Leikert (2023) even assumes a bodily unconscious. I cannot follow such a perspective (see also Lombardi's (2023) well-founded criticism of this view).
9 The thesis of timelessness meets with great resistance, although it seems to me quite plausible: the unconscious is organised symmetrically, i.e. the laws of logic and linear time do not apply. For example, a past event can therefore unconsciously appear as a future event.

Chapter 2

Attempt at a conceptualisation of the nameless

2.1 Some metapsychological considerations

In the following I would like to present my reflections on these phenomenal areas, metapsychologically, theoretically, clinically, methodologically and treatment-technically.

Nameless states are non-psychicised states. The psychic, one of the few "real" laws we have in psychoanalysis, can only arise in a relationship. I.e. we have to look for the starting point of nameless states in (early) disturbances of the interpsychic relationship. How can we think interpsychic dynamics?

2.1.1 Becoming

Let us imagine the following situation: Our child comes running into our bedroom at night and screams in panic: "There's a lion in the room!" We take our child in our arms, frightened. What happens here?

Let's assume that our child's inner states have condensed to such an extent that they could no longer be "dreamed," but have turned into a panic fear. Let us assume that it is an oral anxiety of being eaten, of being torn to pieces. This devastating fear makes the child run to the primary object. That is, we have two levels: the impressions derived from actual experience (what Freud called: "Lebenseindrücke" – "life impressions") and the preconception[1] of a helpful object.

How might the father (we will assume the father for the sake of the mother's relief) experience this situation intrapsychically? Parents are normally deeply unconsciously, lovingly oriented towards their child. This pre-conceptual orientation, which comes to meet the child's expectation, is embedded in the developed psychic apparatus of the object. Thus the father is able to pre-qualify his child's cry, i.e. to perceive in the cry a deep oral anxiety and to hear the cry as a call. Shortened: the cry as a projection of undigested states of the child and the identification of the state by the father. The nocturnal event can thus be understood as a projective identification, discovered by Bion as a basal communication mechanism.

For an observer, projection, similar to drive, comprises source, urge, goal and object. Intrapsychically, the child experiences undigested states that unfold

DOI: 10.4324/9781003434207-3

devastating danger and the expectation of an object, which, however, can no longer be thought in the storm of impressions, but must be sought out in real terms.

The father, who is deeply psychically oriented towards his child, has the ability to identify the projected. To identify here means, and this is very important, to divine/sense within the framework of *his* psychic system. This is the first (transitive) part of identification. The second (intransitive) part of identification is more complicated. To identify with the projected means to become identical with it – as far as possible – *and* to connect with states of one's own unconscious. I.e. I identify my child's fear as an oral anxiety of being eaten, in this identification I become my child, this fear, *and* must connect it with my own deeply unconscious oral fears of destruction.

I understand Bion's "becoming" (e.g. 1965, Chapter 11; 1970, Chapter 3) to mean not becoming the child's anxiety. Rather, "becoming" is the becoming of an anxiety in itself, in which the child's panic fear and the abysses of the object's anxiety are grounded. Anxiety has its own (metapsychological) reality.

If the object were to "only" become the child's fear, the likelihood that it could be helpfully effective is small. For such becoming persists in a distancing and identifying position (see Bion, 1970, 27), both – in Bion's language – K-positions. That is, we must become "anxiety" in order to be able to recognise and name the "evolution" (Bion) of this anxiety in the form of the nocturnal state: "In so far as the analyst becomes O he is able to know the events that are evolutions of O" (Bion, 1970, 27).

The event, we have to know, is the nocturnal anxiety attack of our child. Thus becoming is only possible in a relationship. The state must be common to both. When the father takes his child in his arms and finds the appropriate words, the state has (empirically) "become."

Let us briefly note: Becoming means the becoming of a state (a fear in itself) from which the form that has become has evolved (fear of the lion). If the self is overwhelmed with this process, it needs an object so that this becoming can happen in the relationship.

This is a very complicated process, which is not easy to describe, because we come into areas that occur circularly-paradoxically-aporetically, but we can only describe them chronologically, causally, logically and discursively dissected.

2.1.2 Pre-conception and elements

In my opinion, Bion was the brilliant interpreter of the intuitive Freud. Thus, Bion's concept of pre-conception could have emerged from Freud's intuitive idea of the "primal phantasy" and been interpreted by him in a momentous and profound way. Freud speaks of primal phantasies as

phylogenetically inherited schemata, which, like the categories of philosophy, are concerned with the business of "placing" the impressions derived from actual experience.... Wherever experiences fail to fit in with the hereditary schema, they become remodelled in the imagination.... We are often able to see the schema triumphing over the experience of the individual.

(Freud, 1918b, 119)

A little later Freud writes: "it is hard to dismiss the view that some sort of hardly definable knowledge, something, as it were, preparatory to an understanding, was at work in the child at the time" (ibid., 120).

This definition seems to me to be extremely important: The hereditary schema contains a (supra-individual) knowledge of reality and (psychic) truth, which can very effectively correct disorders and haziness and thus advance mental health. It exists before all experience, but still needs individual experience, which normally has to bow to the creative power of the schemata.

Bion took up this idea with the concept of pre-conception and elaborated on it in many of his writings. In my opinion, the fate of pre-conception is crucial for understanding nameless states.

Bion assumes that there are pre-conceptions which become noticeable as "a state of expectation" (1963, 23), e.g. in the mother and in the new-born a pre-conception of the breast.

However, the pre-conception "breast" is not to be understood as a partial object, but as its complex, relational structure, in which the child, the object and the relationship are laid out, which must then become.

This "unknown expectation" of a mother-child relationship encounters its realisation. The pre-conception must encounter a positive realisation that sufficiently saturates the state of expectation. This saturation must take place through a realisation that has an existence *independent* of the personality (see Bion, 1965, 137).

Bion tries to elaborate this idea:

> I postulate *an α-element version* of a private Oedipus myth which is the means, the pre-conception, by virtue of which the infant is able to establish contact with the parents as they exist in the world of reality. The mating of this α-element Oedipal pre-conception with the realization of the actual parents gives rise to the conception of parents.
>
> (1963, 93; italics BN)

We can extend this description of the Oedipal pre-conception to all pre-conceptions.

I.e. the pre-conception, like the primordial fantasy, exists before all experience. If the expectation is fulfilled, it is *initialised* and *realised*.

At the same time, we can assume with Freud and Bion that there are sensual-bodily impressions and sensations and (external) stimuli that only become psychic elements through the action of a psychic function (α-function), which can combine and be stored in memory. They lend themselves to nocturnal and waking-dreaming. The infant can initially only order these sensual impressions according to pleasure and unpleasure; in too great a quantity they are experienced as displeasure, which can then be excreted to a certain extent. The psychic function of transforming these elements must develop in the relationship to the primary object.

We must now examine this process a little more closely and dissect it artificially. Let us first focus on the infant.

The infant is hungry, i.e. confronted with a swelling of raw, sensual impressions and sensations which have no psychic quality but which nevertheless make themselves agonisingly felt, e.g. in what an observer describes as hunger. Since his self is still immature, they threaten to take on a dissolving, entropic form.

At the same time, the infant has an inherent pre-conception that awakens the expectation of the breast. This pre-conception is probably activated by the sensual sensations and impressions.

I.e. we have raw, non-psychicised elements which, if they spread unhindered, can lead into death-driven threat (entropy), which the infant does not succeed in transforming. At the same time, however, there is a psychic structure that pushes towards the object as an expectation. Although this pre-conception consists of a related structure of α-elements, it still has to be initialised and realised.

This specific constellation now makes it possible for the raw elements to temporarily accumulate in the pre-conceptual structure.[2] Loosely formulated: The expectation, activated by raw sensations and stimuli, captures the same and temporarily holds them together. Thus, the expectation of the breast gets a direction and, filled with raw elements, pushes towards the object. I.e. the pre-conception filled with raw elements is to be understood psycho-somatically. The expectation is α-elementally structured; the embedded elements are raw, sensual sensations.

Now we have to add the object. The object, the mother, is also oriented in pre-conceptual expectation, awaiting her child. But she has a psychically developed apparatus. Thus she has a different access to self-states and is able to order inner and outer impressions. But she too has to deal, perhaps not with raw, but with new sensual sensations and impressions, even if these are given a certain order in primary maternity.

She hears the cry of her child. Involved in the infant's pre-conception are the raw sensual sensations that enable the mother to pre-qualify her child's state. She hears the cry as a call. (It is interesting that parents who have children with severe autistic disorder, in whom we suspect a severe disorder of the pre-conception breast, do not feel called...; see Nissen, 2015.)

Another important aspect now comes into play: The pre-conceptions are to be understood objectally, i.e. the expectation of self, object and relationship that become in the realisation. The pre-conceptions of mother and child are complementary to each other: mother – child – mother-child relationship. In this complementarity, the becoming of the state is prepared.

In an intermediate summary, it can be stated that in the pre-conception there is α-elementary and objectal structure in which the raw sensations and stimuli can accumulate. This unrealised, unsaturated pre-conception is thus to be thought psycho-somatically.

I First clinical illustration: the hurricane[3]

1   A patient books by telephone in a normal way. She appears as a young woman dressed in student style. She makes hardly any contact, seems uncertain, tries to hide behind a friendliness which is almost embarrassing. She looks disoriented, but instantly takes over the entire waiting room. I straightaway find myself in a raging chaos: Her paraphernalia is everywhere: hat, scarf, gloves, jacket, bag, a pack of cigarettes and coins falling out, coffee mug, etc., are scattered throughout the room. She seems to stay put nowhere, she talks incessantly, without my being able to hear her words. My breathing is constricted, I almost come out with nonsense like: "It really is pretty cold out there," though I cannot remember what season we have and if it really is cold. Suddenly, the patient steps in front of the mirror (that hangs in the waiting room) – and it is quiet, like the eye of the hurricane. When she steps back from the mirror, I almost bundle her into the treatment room and shut the door hastily, as I try to banish the raging chaos.

2   "Inside," it remains calm on the surface. Her eyes flit over my face. Then she spreads out her fragmented mental world: She still bears the name of her father, who she does not know. He had cheated on her mother during pregnancy, after which the mother left and took back her maiden name. My patient did not enjoy her studies, but she completed them. She is hypochondriac, afraid of having breast cancer. She examines her breasts for hours, visits several doctors a day, the fear remains. I start again to perceive, to grasp what is fragmented, to intuit her threatened self, feel that she has no place in a relationship. After her birth she had gone to her grandparents for several months, her mother had "joined the hippies." "Commune, free love, always other men, I was often there – sorry, I forgot my tissues out there!" She jumps up: Struck by fear I want to call, "But you do not need... I have..." She is already in the waiting room.

3   It remains calm, quiet, a moment too long. I know that she is looking at herself in the mirror. She comes back and I ask very directly: "Have you been looking at yourself in the mirror again?" For a split second she looks at me. She admits it. I say: "You are afraid of drowning in all this chaos, of dissolving into the fear. In the mirror you make sure of yourself." She nods, looking briefly at me. She breathes heavily and falls silent. I take her into treatment.

Let us first look at the first paragraph (1): After a "normal" registration by telephone, a young patient appears, at first appearing "inconspicuous." But she does not really make contact, seems uncertain, perhaps hiding behind a (façade-like?) embarrassing friendliness. Then she seems disoriented, a storm breaks out, taking over the whole waiting area, growing into a hurricane. Everything seems fragmented and scattered. There is no longer any sense of a relationship being established, of an encounter. Perceptual functions collapse, words become sounds, the Cs system is attacked, contact with reality is restricted. Physiological stress arises, so massive that the self of patient and analyst have to protect themselves with autistoid and psychosomatic measures (incessant talking as second skin; constricted breathing as somatoform reactions). Then she steps in front of the mirror, calm as in the eye of the hurricane. The whipped-up physiological stress can subside a little; certain orientations and secondary-process functions start up again. I almost physically push her into the treatment room.

How might we understand this scene with the theory presented above? Registering with a psychoanalyst activates complex objectal expectations. In this, hopes for holding and understanding are likely to play a central role, i.e. dimensions that correspond to the pre-conception "breast." But this pre-conceptual structure seems to cease to exist immediately after arriving in the waiting area, a massive decomposing process seizes sensual elements and probably also psychic qualities and conceptualisations: Elements are experienced in a bodily, thing-like and raw way, objectal expectation dissolves into singularities in which the self feels threatened. Raw sensual elements no longer find a place in pre-conceptual structures, but the latter become fragments themselves. So finally the self feels threatened.

I think we are mainly dealing with the breaking forth and releasing of nameless elements. The emergence of nameless states cannot be described as a regressive process; that would be a contradiction in terms: Nameless states are unintegrated, not disintegrated! Unintegrated ones are non-psychicised states that are released. This release tears apart qualified and conceptualised structures and elements, an existential threat spreads. In unintegrated processes, defence mechanisms that have psychic structure and operate accordingly also fail. Defences of nameless processes therefore operate with sensory-self-generated forms, e.g. second-skin formations, autistic/autistoid objects, etc. Disintegrated states, on the other hand, are subject to regressive processes undertaken by the self for reasons of defence in order to stabilise at lower levels. In the regressive, psychic dynamics, in this above all the objectal and the defence, remain perceptible.

Let us do a thought experiment: Suppose the patient had gathered up her belongings before or immediately after the mirror scene and fled the practice. Would this scene ever then have attained any psychological significance for me? I do not think so. I would have hypothetically filed it among my empirical knowledge, kept it at a distance with a word, e.g. "The hurricane patient" or "The waiting room scene," but psychically I would not been able to understand it. It would have remained mysterious and strange in my psyche. But I also would not have been able to forget it. Bion writes that there are people who "experience pain but will not suffer it and so cannot be said to discover it" (1970, 9). Discovering, in this sense, would not have been possible. In my opinion, this actual quality should be of great relevance in many nameless states and be a reason for the permanent presence close to the body.

As I said, I see in the "waiting room scene" above all unintegrated dynamics that also forced remaining hopes into dissolving decay. In my opinion, this perspective is underlined by information that I only received in the course of treatment: Many months later when she for the first time began to grasp the sexual border violations emotionally, I learned in the treatment that she felt that the way to the practice, a densely planted, winding garden path, was like an intimate, seductive concentration/intensification, which put her into a state of great tension. This tension released nameless parts that weakened her self and opened up the way to the traumatic primal scene experiences.

This also makes the next scene (2) more understandable.

"Inside" remains calm on the surface, she makes fleeting contact – and is able to hint at her torn life story, to describe her severe hypochondria. I can perceive something of her threatened self and relationship insecurities. She recounts her first traumatic experiences of separation, stumbles associatively to the hippies and to "free love." Almost immediately, a similar stress spreads as in the waiting area: She runs out, I hasp words.

I understand severe hypochondriasis as an autistoid disorder associated with early separation traumatisation and overwhelming arousal (sexual boundary stretching on the part of mothers; abuse as a self-object; unpredictable upheavals in relationships, etc.). I had this knowledge at my disposal when I managed to sense the patient.

If we understand the silence in front of the mirror as a certain reintegration, the patient might have succeeded in feeling herself again, in making contact in the treatment room (her eyes flit over my face) and in communicating. In parallel, I find my way back to a certain understanding, i.e. I also recognise the patient: Encounter and expectation of a relationship become possible. After this objectal movement, she associates overstraining situations (traumas, sexual boundary stretching). Now, does the objectal encounter create the stress that still finds expression in the associations, or do these associations create the stress that is then acted out? In either case, the stress takes on dissolving forms; the patient must mirror herself.

In the third scene (3), the specific calm that is "audible" in the waiting area helps me. With it, I am certain that the patient is looking at herself again in the mirror. For me it is ad hoc, evident that this is a securing of the self. This evidence is not yet a becoming, since becoming can only be in relationship. My question as to whether she looked at herself in the mirror leads my evidence into the shared presence. A presentative symbol has arisen for the salvation of the self (mirroring), which becomes a terminus technicus. This psychic reality, the threat to the self, is only in the constituting relationship: She looks at me, recognises me as an object. I have grasped her; she feels recognised and senses an object that she strives to recognise. The following interpretation, which knows more than I consciously grasped at the time, still names anxiety, dissolution and self-assurance. I do, however, feel that the patient can hardly hear the words. She seems rather to have been contacting her remaining hope that there is an object that is trying to understand her. I experience this as an indicative change of direction: If the hope of a containing object has not been completely destroyed, if the patient is in the first session of an interview in a position to feel the hope, a holding and containing object relationship can probably be built up in treatment. Then I have the belief that the severe hypochondriacal autistoid organisation can be worked on.

2.1.3   Moment of presence

In the last paragraph of the clinical example, the presence moment was already introduced, with which I try to conceptualise Bion's O (see also Stern, 2004: present moment). The O stands for the becoming, or being, of the psychic, from which conceptions and thoughts of psychic phenomena then arise, which become sensually noticeable by their secondary qualities. The psychic itself cannot be grasped sensually:

> The point that demonstrates the divergence most clearly is that the physician is dependent on realization of sensuous experience in contrast with the psychoanalyst whose dependence is on experience that is not sensuous. The physician can see and touch and smell. The realizations with which a psycho-analyst deals cannot be seen or touched; anxiety has no shape or colour, smell or sound. For convenience, I propose to use the term "intuit" as a parallel in the psychoanalyst's domain to the physician's use of "see", "touch", "smell", and "hear".
> (Bion, 1970, 7)

Later, Bion concretises: The presence of O "… can be recognized and felt, but it cannot be known" (1970, 30). O cannot be known, but its presence can be grasped:

> Thoughts have as their background realizations that are sensible: anxiety, fear, sex can be thought about only when O has evolved to a point where it

is apprehensible in sense and has become amenable to transformations in K. Anxiety is "known" by its secondary qualities. Yet no one has any doubt about anxiety or about "feeling" the reality, though what is felt is sensations associated with anxiety and not anxiety itself.

(1970, 35)

In my opinion, this view corresponds completely with Freud's understanding. Freud wrote:

The unconscious is the true psychical reality; in its innermost nature it is as much unknown to us as the reality of the external world, and it is as incompletely presented by the data of consciousness as is the external world by the communications of our sense organs.

(Freud, 1900a, 613)

Freud goes on to ask: "How are we to arrive at a knowledge of the unconscious? It is of course only as something conscious that we know it, after it has undergone transformation or translation into something conscious" (1915e, 166).

In my view, however, we must distinguish between processes in which the psychic is felt and intuited and the perception of the presence of the psychic (O), i.e. the event in which it appears. In the analytic process we sudden0ly ("mirroring" in the example) or insidiously sense the unknown, must be able to wait for the moment in which it becomes apparent, that is, the moment in which it shows itself in presentia, in statu nascendi, for in absentia or in effigie (see Freud, 1912b, 1912e, 1913c, 1914g) it cannot be grasped.

But how are we to grasp the moment of presence if it cannot be known? It must be perceived. We are thus approaching one of the most difficult, unsolved problems not only of psychoanalysis, of consciousness.

Freud does not always seem clear to me on the question of consciousness.[4] But I think, and this is also how I understand Bion, that with Freud it makes sense to distinguish between two forms of consciousness: On the one hand, the system Cs, which, connected with the Pcs and also the Ucs, can recur to functions such as secondary process, reality principle, rational-logical, chronological and spatial thinking and rehearsal action (Freud: "Probehandeln"; "experimental kind of acting"); on the other hand, a perceptual consciousness (Pcpt-Cs), in which there is pure perception without processing by the system Cs.

The systems Cs, Pcs, and Ucs (consciousness, the preconscious and the unconscious) are already divorced, with censorships already established between them. Freud makes it very clear what this systemic valorisation means: "... the existence of the censorship between the *Pcs.* and the *Cs.* teaches us that becoming conscious is no mere act of perception, but is probably also a *hypercathexis*, a further advance in the psychical organization" (1915e, 193f; italics BN). This systemic consciousness is wrested from the undifferentiated matrix and is a higher organisation. Bion notes that at the beginning of life, with reference to Freud: "The limited consciousness defined by Freud, that I am using to define a rudimentary infant consciousness, is not associated with an unconscious. All impressions of the self are of equal value; all are conscious" (Bion, 1962a, 309). This "consciousness produces 'sense-data' of the self, but that there is no alpha-function to convert them into alpha-elements and therefore permit of a capacity for being conscious or unconscious of the self" (Bion, 1962a, 308f).[5]

It is a pure perception consciousness that notices internal and external impressions and sensations without perceiving the *psychic* qualities. Whether there can be such a pure perception consciousness without the qualitative divorce of pleasure-unpleasure remains to be seen. However, the basal qualities pleasure-unpleasure are of utmost importance since they are linked to the motoric and result in turning away from (expulsion, avoidance, withdrawal, flight, etc.) or turning towards (creation, production, change, search, etc.). I assume that this pure perception consciousness exists throughout life. It remains as a perceptual modality even after the α-function has been established. This means that this pure perception consciousness can also exercise its function when the separation of the mental systems has taken place.

We have thus found a way to understand how the psychic can be perceived, but cannot be known: Pure perception consciousness can grasp the psychic state when the reflexive ego is momentarily suspended. More precisely: There are states of pure perception in which the systems Cs, Pcs, Ucs do not interfere with their functions and regularities.

If the primary object is in a sufficiently good maternal state and the infant is sufficiently frustration-tolerant, a psychic reality (and psychic truth) shows itself in the moment of presence in clarity and unambiguity, but not fixed, but floating. I.e. the elements are psychically qualified and self, object and relation are initialised and realised, but have yet to become, since there is no quality and no systemic divorce in pure perception consciousness. A paradoxical, aporetic situation.

The psychic reality that reveals itself has indeed unfolded in the course to the moment of presence forebodingly between two personalities and in their relationship, and has found a pre-qualification. This pre-qualification,[6] which is also grounded in intuition, creates a loose, temporary connection between the elements that stabilise the expectation of the encounter (Faith; F). But this pre-qualification dissolves again in the moment of presence, since here reality shows itself as a floating potentiality. But without the pre-qualification, perceiving the state would become more difficult (see also endnote 6). It is important that memory and desire are not given any ordering power here. In the worst case, pre-determinating processes could occur (see Bion, 1965, 137). I.e. in the moment of presence, a psychic reality cannot show itself per se (here I thus deviate from Bion), but only an evolution of the psychic out of the relationship, even if it is there in pure form (in itself), not contaminated by secondary qualities. The reality that enters ultimately remains asymmetrically that of the child/patient[7].

I.e. in the moment of presence, only an evolution of a psychic reality shows itself, however not sensually and qualitatively, but "in itself." This leaves open the question of whether "anxiety in itself," as in Bion, is to be assumed as O, as ultimate reality (e.g. 1965, 140; 1970, 26). I assume, however, that in the moment of presence the couple experiences a reality in itself, that is, one that temporarily subjugates the participants in a powerful way.

In the "hurricane example," the patient is swept away by a fear of dissolution that carries me away. There is no question: The fear has taken hold of both of us, we experience dissolution anxiety, which at its core remains the patient's fear. In the moment of presence, when mirroring is discovered as a safeguard of the self against dissolution, this reality is undeniably there and can be differentiated: drowning in all this chaos, dissolving into the fear, making sure of yourself.

At this point we can define pre-conception/conception more precisely: Pre-conception is the expectation of self, object and relation. In this objectal structure, a pre-qualified state (e.g. dissolving fear) emerges via raw elements, which refers to a psychic reality in itself. But this is not enough; for in the objectal dimension of expectation, being known, holding, understanding and love are included (see Bion's reflections on the act of faith, which belongs to the system O (1970, 34ff), but is in O, in my opinion, absent; see Nissen, 2015). That is, in the moment of presence, a psychic reality (an anxiety) shows up in itself, but it is secured (geborgen) in faith. The realisation of self, object and relation is circularly interdependent with the realisation of psychic states (e.g. love, anxiety).

Only in this way can fear experience its sublation, for which Bion describes two forms: On the one hand, states are made bearable, e.g. fear of death into bearable, held fright (Bion, 1962a), and, on the other hand, states are transformed (Bion, 1963), e.g. ghastly hunger into blissful contentment, even if both states exist eo ipso (see Nissen, 2021).

Here the different fates of conception formation now also become visible: For the infant or for the patient suffering from nameless states, the realisation of the objectal dimensions with their libidinous qualifiers is paramount: the existence of the relationship, the object and the self, being known, feeling love, support, understanding and states made bearable (terror instead of dissolution; blissful contentment; see case example in which the patient felt less the content than the objectal dimension). The object with its psychic apparatus, on the other hand, can connect the states associated with unpleasure/pain and threat in the conception and can use them in future encounters.

2.1.4 Transformation into the presentative

The presence moment occurs in pure perception consciousness. Thus it can only be a "moment," since this form of perception is not permanent and the system Cs naturally comes into effect again. Concealment is therefore inherent in the presence moment. If the presence moment were not sublated, it would become traumatic.

But when the system Cs comes into effect again, psychic qualities can be perceived. Freud puts forward the thesis that the consciousness functions as "a sense-organ for the perception of psychical qualities" (1900a, 615; see also 1915e). This definition is also central for Bion (see e.g. 1962, 86; 103; 1965, 115; 1970, 28). Qualities do not exist in the Pcpt-Cs; these are only perceived in the

Cs. The psychic-qualified elements are then fixed and connected in the realised conception – thus stabilising the conception. An O→K transformation.

But the system Cs is connected to the Pcs and Ucs and is more highly organised. The perception of psychic qualities is thus subject to requirements of the psychic systems. These requirements not only perceive the complexity of the moment of presence, but also order and shape it. Complexity means in simple terms that "because of immanent constraints in the elements' connective capacity, it is no longer possible at any moment to connect every element with every other element" (Luhmann, 1995, 24), meaning that elements can only be linked selectively. If the system Cs comes into its own again, it qualifies elements in this complexity as psychic and creates constant connections. The perception of psychic qualities is thus to be understood as a selective and reductive one: Elements are selected and delimited in their meaning.

More than that, the ordering of the elements must satisfy the Pcs and Ucs systems if the conception is to be a psychically stable and significant one. Here we must conceive of psychic qualification as conscious presentation, as Freud defines it: "the conscious presentation comprises the presentation of the thing plus the presentation of the word belonging to it" (1915e, 201). That is, the conception that sublates the moment of presence must rest in the psychic systems.

It gets even more complicated:

In conception, self, object and relation have become. This having become must be taken into account. The self is inescapably connected to the object in the relationship. In my opinion, the systems theorist Luhmann can help us again here:

> We speak of "penetration" when a system *makes* its own *complexity* (and with it indeterminacy, contingency, and the pressure to select) *available for constructing another system*. Precisely in this sense social systems presuppose "life". Accordingly, *interpenetration* exists when this occurs reciprocally, that is, when both systems enable each other by introducing their own already constituted complexity into each other. In penetration, one can observe how the *behaviour* of the penetrating system is co-determined by the receiving system … In interpenetration, the receiving system also reacts to the *structural formation* of the penetrating system, and it does so in a twofold way, internally and externally. This means that greater degrees of freedom are possible in spite (better: because!) of increased dependencies. This also means that, in the course of evolution, interpenetration individualizes behaviour more than penetration does.
>
> (Luhmann, 1995, 213)

That is, self and object mutually make complexity available to each other, so that an objectal, psychically qualified conception can emerge, which, although arising in the greatest dependence, allows for higher degrees of freedom.

Bion tries to grasp this process with the term "constellation":

> The facilitation of "constellation" must in turn be seen as a step in the process of at-one-ment (the transformation O → K). In practice this means not that the

analyst recalls some relevant memory but that a relevant constellation will be evoked during the process of at-one-ment with O, the process denoted by transformation O → K.

(1970, 33)

In an important footnote he specifies the term: "I use the term 'constellation' to represent the process precipitating a constant conjunction" (1970, 33).

The conception, although a reduction of complexity, is to be thought of as complex: In it, self, object and relation have become; it thus emerges *interpsychically*, and in it, selective psychic elements that must satisfy *all intrapsychic* systems are constantly connected.

By definition, a conception understood in this way, grounded in all systems, can never be fully grasped. And yet, in order for the presence moment to be sublated, the incomprehensible complexity must be condensed, at the same time preserved. Bion introduces the following idea:

> The abstraction, or formulation, of a generalization consists in the naming of a new entity. What has been regarded as a dynamic state in which elements of a realization are abstracted selectively to form an abstraction, generalization or, more abstractly still, an algebraic calculus, should be regarded as the mating of a pre-conception with a realization to form a conception and thus a reformulation: the reformulation is a naming of the total constellation of pre-conception and conception to prevent the loss of the experience by dispersion or disintegration of its components. The process known as abstraction is related to notation (as described by Freud) and an enlargement of memory.
>
> (Bion, 1963, 85)

However, in my opinion, the term reformulation summarises too many different processes, namely, the first naming of the presence moment up to the formation of thoughts (see below). In my opinion, the sublation of the presence moment can be well illustrated with the theory of Susan Langer (1942), who created the term presentational symbol. It captures a state that is so complex that it can only be preserved in the presentative symbol, never fully described discursively. The complexity of the moment of presence is thus sublated in the presentational symbol.

We can illustrate this process in our example: The complexity of chaos, dissolution, demise, survival, self-preservation cannot be grasped. The first presentative symbol "mirroring" is for both participants a word-presentation with an immense psychic "substructure" that could not have been unconscious until then. This experience can (hopefully) submerge into the unconscious as a thing presentation later in the analytic process. In the presentative name "mirroring," elements are presentatively qualified and interconnected. The naming that is done in the following, more discursive interpretation, specifies this terminus technicus, but with considerable loss: Drowning, dissolving, self-securing are central components in the created conception, but felt too narrowly.

We can already note at this point three characteristics of the presentative that result from the derivation and are important for therapeutic practice. The sublation into the presentative includes the discovery of the psychic reality that occurred in the moment of presence, is a creation of the couple that is to be sought in the relationship and its interpsychic dynamics as well as in the selective reduction of complexity, and has a supra-effective quality, i.e. the psychic reality confronts the actors as an independent entity.

The discovery of psychic reality involves the dissolution of connections between elements and the floating of a new relation, as well as the repositioning of relationship, self and object. Although this moment is not fixed, it is a discovery behind which one cannot go back. The determination of this open potentiality is a creative act of the couple, but in its asymmetry the state of the self becomes recognisable above all. The creative act, however, is not entirely within the sovereignty of the participants, since the discovery and naming brings forth a reality to which they also have to "submit."[8]

2.1.5 From presentative to representative

Freud developed a model in his writings (see seventh chapter of the Interpretation of Dreams; the central metapsychological writings between 1914 and 1917) that describes this early development. A baby is confronted with internal stimuli which he experiences with unpleasure and which we call hunger. The mother breastfeeds him; an experience of satisfaction ("Befriedigungserlebnis") occurs. When further sensations of hunger occur, he switches to the "hallucinatory cathecting of the memory of satisfaction" (Freud, 1900a, 598); he sucks his thumb or comforter.

This hallucinatory wish fulfilment can be experienced for a time as indistinguishable from the real, experienced event of satisfaction ("perceptual identity"; 1900a, 566). But the hardness of reality will teach him; unpleasure increases. A tension between the experience of real satisfaction (at the breast) and a hallucinatory replication arises. "Such hallucinations, however, if they were not to be maintained to the point of exhaustion, proved to be inadequate to bring about the cessation of the need or, accordingly, the pleasure attaching to satisfaction" (1900a, 598).[9] "The bitter experience of life must have changed this primitive thought-activity into a more expedient secondary one" (Freud, 1900a, 566).

This simplest developmental psychological model makes clear what the central demands on the infant's immature mental system are: abandonment of the omnipotence active in hallucinatory wish fulfilment; development of a secondary apparatus that modifies primitive thought activity. But Bion, in my opinion, now goes a step beyond Freud, since he emphasises the recognition of an object that has an existence *independent* of the personality (see Bion, 1965, 137) and on which the self is existentially dependent. That is, the absence of the object is to be thought so that conception can become thought (see Bion, 1963, Chapter 8; also Levine, 2013, 47).

The conception of the "breast" evolves in the relationship. Although it is a constant connection, it is stable for the infant only in the presence of the object;

otherwise it quickly proves unstable. In the absence of the object, he can only resort to hallucinatory, thus self-generated sensations. However, this hallucinatory wish fulfilment cannot permanently defy the bitter experience of life.

The recurring, pressing hunger activates a preconception "breast" that is based on a positive realisation experience. This preconception emerged from a conception in which the present object and the relationship to it were recognised, in which libidinous states became and in which primarily experiences of satisfaction were qualified. That is, neither was the absent object conceptualised nor were the raw elements associated with threat/terror and absence sufficiently qualified. The non-conceptualised "absent breast" is now associated with sensations and affective discharges that accompany hunger. These raw elements threaten the self and pre-conceptual, objectal hopes.

From these tensions, absent-present object and threatening, insufficiently qualified elements-qualified satisfactions, work demands on the early self arise, possibly corresponding to a "primitive thinking" to which Bion alludes:

> Nevertheless there are grounds for supposing that a primitive "thinking," active in the development of thought, should be distinguished from the thinking that is required for the use of thoughts. The thinking used in the development of thoughts differs from the thinking required to use the thoughts when developed.
>
> (1963, 35)

This primitive thinking, however, needs an object that is able to identify these states in itself *and* to experience itself as the absent, threatening object. I.e. it must become the object that subjects the infant to these threatening and unthinkable states. It must therefore experience itself as the object that imposes such states on the child to whom it is deeply attached in love. Resistance arises against this imposition, which runs completely counter to us, because we have to become an object that we do not want to be and yet are. But in these resistances, separation and separateness and the otherness of the object lie dormant. That is, the primary object is separate from the child and in this separateness becomes the evil object, not only in perception but in the psychic system really. But these are precisely the factualities that it takes to be able to form the thought "absent object."

So the object must not only identify the child's experience of being traumatically-destructively threatened and must identify with this experience and connect it to its own unconscious fears of annihilation, but *become the annihilating object*! This is the decisive extension of identification, which produces other, strong resistances. And yet this becoming must occur. But this becoming can now only become in the relationship to the child.

When this succeeds, a paradoxical situation occurs: In these processes, the child experiences not only that potentially traumatic nameless states spread, but that the conception of a "present breast" disintegrates. I.e. with Winnicott, his going on being is threatened. But it experiences at the same time (in whatever modalities) an object that is capable of becoming truly "evil" and can acknowledge it. But an object that remains perceptibly loving and can acknowledge its "being evil" cannot be evil, but proves to be loving-understanding. Thus, tension can become difference, in which the absent object is the non-present object.

In this way, a mosaic of different conceptions emerges, which relate to each other, reset themselves preconceptually, reconceptualise themselves, etc. The resulting interconnectedness becomes a network. The resulting network becomes increasingly stable, forms constant connections and thus establishes a boundary. A thought emerges, i.e. a complex conception that survives the absence of the object. The thought receives a "name" (however, this name is experienced by the infant). In names phenomena are connected; at the same time phenomena can be felt to belong and the connection of phenomena is protected from disintegration (see Bion's discussion of the name "dog," 1963, 87ff). With this constant connection, meaning can be explored: "On the PS ↔ Dep operation depends the delineation of the whole object: on the successful operation of ♀♂ depends the meaning of the whole object" (1963, 90).

2.1.6 Thinking the thoughts

A new work requirement emerges, namely, to develop a thinking that can think thoughts. In the process, the primitive "thinking" which was more a passive-endured dynamic is subsequently transformed into an active-omnipotent one: The object is used.

With the thought, relationship and an independent object have arisen for the subject, which can be "good" and "bad," present and absent, and has its own inner world with its own motives, etc. The object is used. A process of separation has grown out of a dependency, in which the dimension of separateness and independence emerges, which, as seen, increases degrees of freedom. This development is there as a potentiality and must now be developed.

In my opinion, Winnicott's reflections on the use of the object can help here, even if he thinks from a completely different concept of the object. The central question is how the object can be thought of as an object, i.e. as an independent being.

> When I speak of the use of an object, however, I take object-relating for granted, and add new features that involve the nature and the behaviour of the object. For instance, the object, if it is to be used, must necessarily be real in the sense of being part of shared reality, not a bundle of projections. It is this, I think, that makes for the world of difference that exists between relating and usage.
>
> (Winnicott, 1969, 712)

This is how I think the famous paradox must be read: "The baby creates the object but the object was there waiting to be created and to become a cathected object" (1969, 713). That is, in the focal point of this dynamic, the object is there to be created. In the development of a thought, the infant's omnipotence turned into passive

helplessness and existential dependence. The thought can be understood as the discovery that the object exists outside the self:

> This thing that there is in between relating and use is the subject's placing of
> the object outside the area of the subject's omnipotent control, that is, the sub-
> ject's perception of the object as an external phenomenon, not as a projective
> entity, in fact recognition of it as an entity in its own right.
>
> (1969, 713)[10]

A step on the way to the reality principle, but also to the use of phantasy. For this,
the object is created in order to acknowledge its "non-creation."

This creation takes place through the destruction of the object. The object survives the destruction and does "not retaliate" (1969, 714). The destruction and
retrieval of the object are omnipotent processes. Paradoxically, the object is destroyed not only because it exists outside omnipotent control, but also because the
destruction places it outside omnipotent control (see Winnicott, 1969, 713). Thus
it becomes possible to conceive dependence and separateness. But this process is
made possible by the fact that the object has recognised itself as the destructive
one. I.e. two things: The object was able to acknowledge its destructive parts and
to sublate them in such a way that a thought could emerge for the child. In this way,
the child's threatening (annihilation) fear is given a place and a reality – and can
be led from the passive-threatening into the active-raging. The desire to destroy the
object has thus found a reason ("You, object have threatened me") and a safeguard;
for the object could sublate its destructive parts in itself and thus save the relationship. I.e. the use of the object takes place in a framework that makes the dynamic
possible.

This figure of creation and destruction (a fantastic game of Fort-Da) differentiates not only the self-object relationship but thus allows a view of the self and the
object from its third perspective. If this fantasy detaches itself from omnipotence
and the object becomes an external one that I need, the object that is now absent was present before and will be there again, not vengeful but understanding.
A thought can be thought.

2.2   The absence of realisation

The above basic theoretical attempt enables a model for thinking about the psycho-
genesis of the nameless.[11]

Hunger releases unpleasant, raw sensual sensations for the infant that activate
the pre-conception "breast" (as defined). The sensations temporarily attach themselves to this expectation, thus helping the mother to hear and pre-qualify the cry
as a call. If the pre-conceptions of mother and child meet with a sufficiently good
realisation, a conception emerges in which mother, child and relationship as well
as mental states and qualified elements emerge. The elements link together in the
conception; the conception is stabilised by the elements.

If the pre-conception filled with raw sensual elements does not meet with a sufficiently good realisation, no conception can arise. The initialisation and realisation of the α-elementary pre-conception fails to occur, as does the qualification of the sensual elements into psychically significant (α-elements). The α-elementary expectation is therefore not given any meaning and, as an unrealised schema, does not offer any connection and linking possibilities. A self-repair, as Freud postulated for the schema, becomes increasingly difficult.

The emerging self is confronted with a flood of non-psychicised elements, but what is decisive is the fate of the unrealised pre-conception; it is the core of the nameless. Schematically, three dynamics could be distinguished: misconception, pre-determination, nameless states in the narrower sense.

2.2.1   Misconception

Bion writes:

> [the term "hallucination"] must be distinguished from an illusion or delusion because both these terms are required to represent other phenomena, namely those that are associated with pre-conceptions that turn to conceptions because they mate with realizations that do not approximate to the pre-conceptions closely enough to saturate the pre-conception, but closely enough to give rise to a conception or mis-conception.
>
> (1965, 137)

In these states, objectal hopes remain existent, but are not fulfilled by the misconception. A vicious circle comes into being, since the formation of subsequent preconceptions is made more difficult, possibly even impossible, so that the development and differentiation of conceptions can fail to take place. If such a process continues, the violent attempts described by Bion (1959) to achieve relief through excessive discharges and to encounter a saturating realisation are likely to occur. Since, however, the object is not sufficiently realised due to the deficient formation of the conception, these "projections" do not take place into an object that has been there but into a "preconception" that has not emerged from a conception. The growing number of elements that cannot be connected puts a strain on the object-expecting structure, which begins to become fragile. The resulting states are characterised by extreme physical tension and disruption, by an imminent unintegration of the self.

2.2.2   Pre-determination

If it is not possible to form a conception leading to contact with reality and to the principle of reality, the existence of a reality independent of the personality cannot be tolerated. The intrapsychic "non-reality" must be elevated to "reality," and reality must be immediately subdued to this non-reality. Not only does an inability to represent emerge, but also an inability to be (see Bion, 1970, 18). No misconception arises, but a self-generated state:

> The pre-conception requires saturation by a realization that is *not* an evacuation of the senses but has an existence independent of the personality. The hallucination arises from a pre-determination and requires satisfaction from (a) an evacuation from the personality and (b) from conviction that the element is its own evacuation.
>
> (Bion, 1965, 137)

In the hallucination, the preconception becomes a pre-determination, "satisfied" by self-generated and ejected sensual elements. The object becomes at best a rival; meaningfully psychic becomes a pre-psychic sense impression. This also means, however, that the α-elements of the preconception are stripped of their psychic dimension. It is the return to the pleasure-unpleasure/pain series.

> In the domain of hallucinosis the mental event is transformed into a sense impression and sense impressions in this domain do not have meaning; they provide pleasure or pain. In this way the unsense-able mental phenomenon is transformed into a beta-element which can be evacuated and reintroduced so that the act yields, not a meaning, but pleasure or pain.
>
> (Bion, 1970, 37)

In these dynamics, transformation processes are permanently taking place in which psychically significant things are reset into β-elementary sense impressions. The unrealised breast as well as the stripped elements are psychically nameless. This namelessness is frequently hidden behind a camouflaged, highly efficient and functional façade, but can be observed through the dynamic movements. Bion points out how important the analytical attitude of no memory, no desire is in such processes, first, because there is a psychic need for conceptions and reality, and, second, because concealments can be almost perfect.

Pre-determined states hardly attain psychic quality. Yet primitive projective mechanisms remain at work in these dynamics. In hallucinosis, a reference to reality persists in denial (in Freud's sense) and is perverted to demonstrate the superiority of self-created "reality." Therefore, evacuating mechanisms and pleasure-unpleasure remain in their right. Nameless states in the narrow sense have lost such reference.

2.2.3 Nameless states in the narrower sense

Nameless states in the narrower sense differ significantly from the two aforementioned dynamics.

The non-realisation of the pre-conception does not allow self, object and relation to become and the psychic reality of being held and being understood not to be there. The nameless cannot be put into words; emptiness, nothingness, nullification are attempts at paraphrasing. The going on being is suspended, cannot be experienced retrospectively as continuity. The hope for an understanding object does not exist, thus projective identification also fails, finally every form of primitive projection (expulsion, evacuation etc.). Thus there are also no desperate attempts to reach the object or to create a reality of one's own with sensual elements. The void, the nothingness represent the "traumatic" noxe, are "hidden away" or encapsulated – and yet present as mute, dark, distant, hidden actual.

II Clinical illustration: Severe depression

I had to experience a state that I think corresponds to such experiences in the treatment of a severe depression[12]:

A severely depressed patient tried (in an agonising phase, lasting weeks) to let me know what it was like inside him: "Everything is frozen, 'All life is dead', 'I feel nothing, nothing at all', 'It's destruction', 'It is there but I cannot describe or communicate it.'"

For me it was virtually impossible to understand, to grasp what he was saying. Empathically to grasp what was going on inside him was hardly possible. Empathy became a strenuous undertaking, to imagine actively what it must look like inside a person in whom all is dead and who is no longer able to communicate it. It was also evident that none of my sentences really got through to him or touched him. A tremendous pressure arose; I was afraid of the sessions because I knew I couldn't do anything and the leaden feeling of oppressiveness weighed down on everything, on me, too.

Yet he came to every session, always on time (it wasn't always like that!) as if he wanted to draw me unconsciously into his world. In one of the sessions, it was the last one of the week, he suddenly said: "It's as if an invisible power is sucking all mental life out of me." (Note the "as if"!) Instantly I had the feeling that an invisible power in me was pressing all psychic life into an atomic core and that nothing psychic could escape this dark core. My body was seized with panic. I was sure that it was impossible to escape this black hole and to flee this state.

I said to the patient: "It must be awful to feel like that" and ended the session. I noticed that he had listened attentively, for the first time during this phase. After the session the "dark core" vanished but I remained dazed and shocked for the rest of the day. At the same time I didn't want to be reminded of it and avoided thinking about this "incident."

The following weekend I was busy doing something, and this state reoccurred out of the blue. I tried to explain it to my wife. She understood absolutely nothing. I couldn't explain it and knew that it was impossible. For the first time I understood depressive captivity, depressive lock-in: All psychic life collapses and intrapsychic as well as interpsychic communication fails. Neither depression nor panic is communicable, indeed even non-communicability is not communicable. The self feels threatened by dissolution and annihilation; the objects degenerate to a two-dimensional non-existence. For the first time I realised that such depression consists of two plus one components. On the "inside" there is (a) mental death and (b) the impossibility of communicating this state. Only the failure of all psychic communication leads to the autistoid closing of this state and to unbearableness. The other component is on the "outside," the objects degenerate, are lost in not understanding, become unfamiliar and remote.

The state, which I had only moments to endure, was so unbearable that I could not imagine continuing to live with it: "sending the body to death which has already happened to the psyche" (Winnicott, 1974, 106). [13]

I could imagine that this state captures something of the experience in which a mental death, a nullification, occurs and a complete loss of object takes place. At the beginning of life, however, it might be even more unimaginable: A self does not come into being and the object does not become – and life and being loved do not attain psychic reality. It is important to understand this state as a nameless core and not to confuse it with the accompanying panic, or the flooding with raw sensual impressions and sensations that push deathly into dissolution.

Since projection fails for this core complex, the way in which the raw elements are dealt with must also be different from that in the misconception and the pre-determined states. These elements, which do not acquire a psychic quality and pulsate unintegrated, unchanged, are perceived as excitations that cannot be expelled as non-psychic elements, but instead cluster around the nameless core. In the example, the core would be the depressive dead, the arousal the panic (panic here is the term of a more mature self).

These states of excitement threaten in a death drive-like way (entropy) the self that has survived. This intolerability often leads to a perverse dynamic in which the passive being at the mercy is transformed into an active form; i.e. passivity is replaced by activity. The excitement is then sought for its own sake; i.e. the passive experience of agonising excitement is actively sought and potentiated, not infrequently preferred to human relationships, but thus again subjugating the self.

Despite this perverse substitution, the threat is never really averted; the entropy of the raw elements, which have a debilitating effect like free radicals, as well as the nameless core prevent any form of change. Therefore, autistoid mechanisms are additionally activated almost regularly, which are supposed to dampen the threat and – since they are self-generated – are always available. These mechanisms can take many forms, as the work of recent years has shown (for an overview, see Nissen, 2008; Rhode, 2018).

These different mechanisms can be well illustrated by the "hurricane example": The torrent of released elements floods the entire antechamber and must be banished by an autistoid measure, mirroring as a second skin. The nameless core of hypochondria is only indirectly accessible and named as a dissolution. Hypochondria fulfils many functions, e.g. substitute capsule for the released nameless, but is also a form of channelling the indeterminate, pulsating excitement. The free, raw excitations are repeatedly channelled into the hypochondriacal self-examinations, which can take on an intoxicating, even orgiastic quality, but are nevertheless bound in the organ examinations (binding of the entropic danger). Thus the organ examinations become a reservoir for excitations, at the same time an autistoid object: oppressed, palpated, maltreated not much differently than the autistic object, e.g. the spinning top, for the child.

In the nameless in the strict sense, there is no conception (also no predetermination or misconception) and there is no name for the missing conception. Even more, nameless states seem to be non-existent (see Winnicott). I.e. the absence of realisation does not lead to a presentative symbol either – and not even afterwards (nachträglich). Although this is a relatively clearly punched-out area and subsequent developments can still be sufficiently satisfactory, there remains a weakness in central psychological facts of life. Normally, at the moment of presence, when the pre-conceptual breast is realised, central nuclei for dependency and separation are laid, which are differentiated and stabilised in subsequent thought formation. But these foundations do not form and basal insecurities pervade life. In my opinion, one patient described this state very aptly: "It is more a survival than a life."

The nameless core can hardly be sensed intuitively even by a trained observer, but it does eventually show itself. Either a current event occurs that connects with the nameless one and finally leads the patient in treatment. Or indirect phenomena show up in the treatment (such as the absence of resonance and transference), or a dark "background radiation" becomes perceptible, or we catch ourselves "adding" relational and affective dimensions that are not there at all, or we notice the perverse excitement and autistic/autistoid mechanisms. Through this noticing, objectal dimensions can open up and become pre-conceptual hope.

2.3   Clinical-theoretical reflections on the treatment of nameless states

From the basic theoretical considerations and on the basis of the determination of nameless states, I believe that clinical processes can be theoretically understood. I will illustrate this with an example that I have already discussed several times from various points of view (see endnote 3).

III A case study: autistoid perversion

Breakdown and autistoid perversion

The patient was a very intelligent woman, about 40 years old, who had developed, among other things, a perversion: Faeces trigger violent sexual excitement, they are eaten, she smears her whole body with faeces and urine. On two occasions she became seriously infected by these practices, once life-threateningly. The perversion was practised alone, though also with frequently changing other objects, although "the others as persons, as individuals, do not play a role" (patient's words). She frequently allowed herself to be anally penetrated, unprotected, in such states of arousal. For many years, from inflammatory bowel complaints that required frequent visits to the toilet and caused diarrhoea.

Because of an infection, so the narrative, she wasn't ever taken into her mother or father's arm in her first year of life. The narrative can be doubted in its absolutely literal form: The mother must have held her child, even against medical advice. It could be felt that the mother loved her, beamed at her, played with her and laughed.

The perversion became apparent after she met a sex-addicted man, whose sexuality was infused with an extreme death drive quality.

We could regard the psychosomatic symptoms with the Paris School as an expression of psychically unrepresented states.[14] More important, however, is the encounter with the sex-addicted man, whose sexuality was permeated with death instincts. Something was triggered in this encounter, even if the patient could not put it into words. However, it is not a communication from unconscious to unconscious, but an event that I have called "induction" (Nissen, 2014), Moser infection (2021) and Bendetti osmosis (1983). The patient becomes infected, an infection that triggers a reverberation to the nullification in the earliest age. But since the breakdown was not experienced, nothing of the nameless core can be "remembered." What is activated are arousals that the patient almost immediately diverts into a perverse dynamic and, since the dissolving dangers cannot be banished, expands into an autistoid defence: She smears her whole body with faeces and urine – a second-skin formation in the most literal sense.

If the core of the breakdown seemed non-existent, the perversion and the autistoid defence were also psychically non-existent. So they were not discovered in treatment either, whether as shame, disgust, sexual arousal, split-off activity; as suffering, problem, conflict, destruction, hatred, annihilation. Nor did it emerge sensually, for example, in its greasy, stinking features. No echo, no emotional resonance arose in me. When she spoke of the practices, it was as if she was communicating that she had completed some routine task. *If* I thought I sensed anything at all, it was a distant, alien, near-death, objectless lostness.

The emergence of the breakdown in treatment

At the same time the beginning of the analysis was surprisingly lively – a phase of happiness began.[15] The patient very quickly seemed to feel secure and safe in the treatment: When I came to the practice from my office (I have to walk along a small garden path so that patients who come early can see me – this patient always came a few minutes early), she beamed at me. She looked like a toddler who sees the mother and excitedly wiggles her hands and kicks her legs. Although there was no such motoric discharge, her eyes were shining and I had a feeling of deep joy inside me. The treatment was a joyful get-together: we had a similar sense of humour, liked the same things – and the patient was well aware of this.

If I interpreted this happiness or even connected it with "not being held," a moment of "nothingness" arose – before she cheerfully continued. Her descriptions of the perversion or her oppressive forlornness remained equally blanked out, e.g. when she told me, without any psychic or objectal connection, how she used to drive aimlessly through the city at night in her car.

I think we can observe in this dynamic the coexistence of residues of psychically alive world, which have been hypomanically heightened, and psychic non-existence, which do not seem to touch each other.

But there was something crazy about the situation: Analyst and analysand pretend that there was a living, loving, joyful relationship that was sufficient, even fulfilling. There were certainly islands of realised "happiness" in the early life history, but the fundamental facticity was the breakdown of going on being. A past that did not exist as needed seemed to be there, a past that had occurred as a breakdown and continued as nothingness was as non-existent. Psychical mechanisms, such as denial, ego splitting, manic defence, were mixed into non-existent dynamics.

But from the tension between jubilant happiness and nothingness, microcosmic attunements developed between the patient and myself. Thus, these joyful, excited atmospheres produced a guilt-ridden discomfort in me, caused by the fear of acting with and through this entanglement without addressing the nothingness, the nameless. I found no way to bring it into treatment.

But more important were enactments that immediately began to unfold in the relationship. One day, for example, the patient began to avert her gaze when I arrived. She gave me a little smile, lowered her eyes or looked away. I was irritated.

More and more there was an increasing tension in the air which is difficult to describe, an apprehension and fear of a realisation which, at last, culminated in a touch. Instead of sitting on the chair and waiting, the patient had gone to the toilet. When greeting me, she hesitated to shake hands. Her hands were still damp. She was silent. She then said she had wondered about shaking my hand as before the session at home she had had her faeces in her hands. She had washed her hands thoroughly, also using disinfectant, but felt she had to wash her hands again here. For the first time I felt a moment of disgust and inner distancing.

This dynamic can be understood as follows: nothingness, blanked out forlornness, avoiding the gaze, damped hands create cracks in the autistoid perversion, which suddenly appears in its sensual qualities and makes the suspicion unavoidable that something is "there," is "coming," that something "nameless" exists. A tension arises between the sensually perceptible autistoid perversion and the approaching nameless on the one hand and the objectal dynamic on the other, in which the reliability of the object is mildly tested (my irritation; my disgust and distancing).

This tension gives rise to pre-conceptual expectations as well as to pre-monitions of this very nameless. That is, "behind" the perverse excitations and autistoid dimensions, the nameless core complex is approached, i.e. the breakdown that occurred in the early relationship as dying forlornness. While a chronological time vector was still predominant in the happiness phase, it has now been reversed: Without the participants knowing what is in store for them, they move towards "something," while at the same time this event, the moment of presence, comes towards them. In this dynamic, an emerging pre-conceptual expectation directed towards the future dominates.

At the same time, there has to be glimmer of faith (F belonging to O) that the emerging pre-conception can withstand the force of the breakdown that will occur and that forlornness-dying can be rendered harmless – even if there can be no guarantee of this.

So there are two things: the expectation that the nameless will show itself in the moment of presence and the hope that the moment will point to a reality that can have a curative effect.

Presence moment

One day the breakdown showed up and the perverse-autistoid contents poured into a session: The patient indicates that she has practised "it" once again for herself alone in the bathtub and uses a projective identification to communicate this. This led to a presence moment in pure perceptual awareness: The scene was there, the patient, myself and the relationship were there. It is like Schrödinger's cat: in the presence moment, the breakdown is there, but whether it becomes re-traumatising or can be sublated is not decided. A and -A at the same time, but without any quality. What the moment will be will only be revealed nachträglich.

The psychic cannot become if the sublation into the presentational symbol is absent. Without this sublation, the presence moment threatens to become traumatic. In the treatment situation, with the return of the Cs system, it was possible to grasp and name the secondary qualities. For I had discovered how the patient felt in the bath scene: lonely and ceasing to be; how the atmosphere is: freezing cold, only the warmth of the excrement is there; how the excrement tastes: inflammatory, even if this is not a taste. I understand that the men with whom she shares the perversion are not objects, but represent an agglutinated, extended self. And I am certain that death will triumph, that the patient will die very soon. She must have felt the dissolution, the nothingness. I don't remember my words, but I told her what the central emotional qualities were and appended to the interpretation: "you are going to die this way." The interpretation was not a masterpiece. But the patient accepted it. Interdependent with the qualifying of her state, the patient perceived an object that is able to contain and is related to her in a concerned way.[16]

With the basic theoretical considerations, this moment can be looked at a little more closely. In the presence moment, the pre-conceptual expectation is realised: patient, analyst and relationship and a state as reality are there. What has emerged besides the objectale dimension? A dying forlornness that becomes a horrific terror in the presence moment; a dying forlornness that becomes hope for life in Being (Dasein) and Being Known (Erkanntsein) from the object; and a multitude of secondary phenomena that give a name to psychic reality in their subsequent transformation. It is all there at once and simultaneously, not chronologically, not logically, not spatially ordered, but qualityless in time and space.[17] So, dying forlornness next to horrific horror, hope for life next to dying forlornness, all next to a multitude of qualityless elements. From this moment of presence, the qualities, the times (past, present and future) and Euclidean space emerge in the sublation of the present.

The presentative sublation

With the re-entry of the system Cs, the presence moment is concealed and sublated in the presentative. Presentational interpretations should be short, precise and definitional, trusting that the presentational as the complex symbol captures the presence moment. My interpretation, which spoke from me, was too long, addressed too many dimensions, threatened to slip into the "discursive" (Langer). Today I would think that a sentence like "What a terrible, dying forlornness that grips everything" is quite sufficient.

The presentative interpretation should above all give a name to the recognised psychic reality in its being understood in the relationship, but at the same time it must avoid overburdening dimensions (e.g. too decided self-object differentiations). It must bundle the multitude of secondary qualities into one name so that complexity is preserved. The dying forlornness could thus have become a presentational symbol. Such an interpretation is a "transference interpretation"; for it signals: "I (analyst) have recognised your state, see your suffering." An object that sees such suffering understandingly is a present, holding one that will care. In being held and understood, the analysand recognises himself in the object and knows about the object. Therefore, the O→K movement is an intimate and very libidinous one. Analysand and analyst now know what the patient has suffered in the breakdown and is doing in the perverse act. The analyst thus also becomes the keeper of reality and a witness.

A psychic connection is created in which elements are held together, which at the same time makes it possible for new phenomena to be discovered.

The presentational symbol is a discovery: The pair discovers the reality of breakdown and the perversion practised in the bathroom. It is only in the Nachträglichkeit that the scene becomes *psychically* real. At the same time, the naming is a creative act of the pair, e.g. "inflammatory taste." And the pair is subject to the power of the sublation. It is not foreseeable, e.g. how the words will work, what power they will unfold. For the patient, the postscript had become the most important: "you are going to die this way." This sentence paraphrased her breakdown experience, her psychic dying as an infant. With this sentence she knew she had a chance to live.

Nevertheless, the analyst and analysand experience the sublation very differently. The patient (or the child) focuses on the object, on the emerging relationship and on hope (experience of satisfaction). The terror of the nameless has a name, an object is there, hope for life shows itself – all in the presence of the object!

The analyst, apart from the relief that understanding brings, is more dazzled by the horror and terror, is objectally concerned and senses the challenges that emerge even after a successful sublation. Yet both believe themselves in the understood, a reassuring delusion.

Formation of thoughts

The patient experiences the sublation into the presentative almost as a redemption: The hope for an understanding object has been fulfilled; the terror is bound and development shines forth. This conception exists for the patient only in the presence of the analyst, much in the same way that the infant experiences more the satisfactions of the nourishing breast, blocking out the tormenting hunger and the absent breast. The child's hunger, however, was not a traumatic experience; being breastfed can therefore find its way into the "memory systems" (Freud) and subsequently have a hallucinatory effect. But the breakdown was the experience of dying, unthinkable, nameless. The absence of the object (analyst) cannot therefore be bridged hallucinatory, but releases the nameless state. It has not yet been sufficiently stable and securely conceptualised; for conception needs the presence of the object to be conceivable. But a reverberating difference has emerged between non-being and the hope and relief of being able to exist. The breakdown is thus no longer *psychically* non-existent, as it was before the analysis, but has become present as a nameless, non-thinkable horror. It shows itself in sensual-entropic flooding with excitations, in which the found object becomes a re-traumatising one, the absent object of the past.

Absence is experienced as a loss of holding in a very basic sense; not being held threatens dissolution, unintegration. It is important to understand this dynamic in all its force, not from the perspective of a mature ego. Because in such dynamics, the mature modes of functioning that the patient has undoubtedly developed can hardly be activated. She is at the mercy of an event that is similar to the rupture in going on being. In the patient's experience, the analyst has conjured up the horror of the breakdown – and then leaves her alone after the session. This constellation is the reason why suicidal, psychotic and psychosomatic episodes (and sometimes severe somatic diseases; see e.g. Klüwer, 2006) so often follow in such dynamics with the presentational sublation.

It is important to understand these suicidal, psychotic and psychosomatic dynamics as benign progression rather than malignant regression. They express the onset of psychisation and are desperate attempts to give expression to a dissolving experience. If an infant who has experienced a sufficiently good, breastfeeding mother can initially meet pressing sensation with a hallucinatory wish fulfilment that results in a cry as a consequence of persistent hunger pangs, patients who have experienced early traumatisation are confronted with the danger of retraumatisation – and give this danger a non-inadequate expression, a presentability. This presentability can also be understood as a helpless, earliest communication in which an experience is communicated.

Theoretically, this perspective is quite easy to understand, clinically, in treatment not only hardly bearable, but undecidable, aporetic! And this for two reasons: It does not have to be a benign progression; it can also be a malignant, even real dangerous dynamic. We are put into a state that causes us the greatest distress. Those who believe they can save themselves to the safe side (according to the motto: "Not so bad, it's benign progression") not only split off inner states, but also act dangerously with them. Above all, if we do not endure the tension of aporetic not-knowing, we would deprive ourselves of the possibility of sublation in the moment of presence. We need this not-knowing to be able to discover ourselves as a traumatising object!

In the patient this dynamic took on extreme forms, which I was at the mercy of without a safety net or false bottom. A suicidal pull towards death unfolded in separations: "I don't want to kill myself, but it will happen.

I'm afraid, no, in panic, do you understand, Mr. Nissen? It is killing me, I'm powerless" – panic that the death pull will triumph, that patient and analyst are powerless. We both knew how serious it was. Just as I was uncertain whether she would come to the next session, the patient was uncertain whether I would discontinue the treatment and arrange a psychiatric admission, which is what all my colleagues advised. But this termination would probably have become a real retraumatisation. My realisation that I had really become the re-traumatising object for the patient, watching impassively, could be brought into the session. At that moment I was the re-traumatising object and at the same time I was not, because with the naming, the identity had become difference. The suicidal horror ("it will happen!") was – fortunately – banished.

In the transference, it is therefore important to establish oneself not only as an absent object, but also as a threatening, re-traumatising one. Then the states that the patient suffers can be there and interpreted.

These paradox-aporetic dynamics, being the re-traumatising object and in becoming it no longer being it, must be discovered in the relationship in the moment of presence. The patient can discover an object that is annihilating – and discover that the object has recognised this annihilating, and so is not annihilating. This paradoxical form in the presence moment gives a shape and a name to the nameless-traumatic. In this conception, the present, evil object and annihilation are sublated and have become thinkable and can be related to the first conception of the holding object. In this way, a conscious presentation (Freud) arises for the patient, from which the thing presentation can descend into the unconscious and is available there for binocular processing.

In this way, a thought for the patient can emerge from the created conceptions. By being the preserver and witness of the reality of a breakdown, and by being able to acknowledge his involvement in the suicidal dynamics that follow, the analyst can be recognised as a holding and understanding object. The experience could be paraphrased as follows: "You, analyst, know about my breakdown; you, analyst, leave me alone, expose me to the dissolving fears – but you really understand, so it must be that you are good to me, want me to live." The relationship becomes conceivable even in the absence of the object. Times emerge: The analyst becomes an external object that is absent in the present, was there in the past and will be there in the future. The actual timelessness of the breakdown, which submerges self and object and is devastatingly threatening, can become a condition that the patient has. Put simply: The patient no longer *is* fear, but *has* fear. State and relationship become thinkable; the object becomes relatable. This development allowed other dynamics to emerge – object use and thinking required to use the thoughts.

So much for the brief clinical-theoretical illustration. In my experience with breakdown states in the narrower sense, the two presence moments presented, discovery of dying forlornness and autistoid perversion, such as discovery of the absent object as re-traumatising, play a central role. They represent mutative vertices, our "magic weapons" (Strachey, 1934), in nameless states. These vertices subdivide the treatment process: First, a rather long phase in which pre-conceptual hopes emerge and are tested for their viability; presence moment in which this pre-conception is realised; turbulent dynamics (reactive-psychotic, suicidal, psychosomatic-somatoform) in which the re-traumatising of the absent object can be sublated in a presence moment.

Even if this scheme cannot be transference to all nameless states, the erection of a containing structure and an apparatus for thinking developed thoughts are central vertices that must be realised, even if cumulative processes are possible instead of the condensed nodes.

2.4   The nameless in specific disease patterns

Beyond the silent and hidden breakdowns, there are many other nameless dynamics, some of which push themselves "loudly" to the fore, but are nevertheless, or precisely because of this, not recognised.

2.4.1   Hypochondria as an autistoid disorder

I choose hypochondria as an example, which Freud regarded as one of the actual neuroses.[18] Severe hypochondria is a mental illness that is distressing and often tends to become chronic. It is considered by many to be almost untreatable. Yet much is openly in front of us. For example, a patient could say:

I suffer from severe anxiety, I am afraid of having xy cancer, real fear of death. Everything has been medically examined, I also say straight away that I am a hypochondriac, nothing will ever be found, but the fear remains....

The patient says very clearly that he suffers from severe anxiety, fear of death, which he associates with cancer. There is no medical finding. He uses the diagnosis "hypochondria," concludes that the anxiety remains.

Despite the clarity, this message is quite confusing for an adult person: Deathly fear of an incurable cancer for which there are no medical findings, but the certified absence of findings does not reassure; the fear remains.

What does this mean for the object relationship? Many of these patients, who are often successful in their careers, have stable relationships and families, can speak quite objectively and reasonably, so that the contradictory, confusing nature of the statement is not so noticeable. The self-designation "hypochondriac" even conceals, tempts medical professionals to make findings so that patients can "feel reassured."

The patient's message does not reach us, not the severe anxiety, not the confusing, contradictory, nothing becomes accessible to us from his inner-soul world. The failed communication, the absence of the object relationship is perhaps registered, but does not open up any space.

But with this we can get on the track of this disorder. A person comes and says he is afraid of death – and we do not feel this person in his threatened state, we simply do not hear him psychically.

Why can we hear the child crying: "There is a lion in the room," but not the patient? Why do we not succeed in translating the communication into an affective, related one, e.g. "There is a cancer in my soul that wants to destroy me"? Then something would take hold of us.

According to my observations, which as always in the psychoanalytic are based on the smallest of data, in severe hypochondria the realisation of the preconception breast fails even in the earliest mother-child encounters and usually continues cumulatively. Real separation traumas are often present, usually already in the first year of life. These traumatic experiences are almost always encapsulated, but remain present close to the body. In many cases, the father is absent. To make matters worse, the children were often abused as the mother's self-object and there is sexual involvement of the children: e.g. they experience the primal scene, or tenderness is intensified to such an extent that it is experienced as sexually assaultive. This circumstance is significant because the arousals surrounding the encapsulations are heightened by these sexual boundary stretches in such a way that they threaten to overwhelm the personality. Here, autistoid measures are almost regularly taken as a further defence.

Very early on, patients seem to have withdrawn hope in an understanding, containing object, so that interpsychic projective mechanisms (e.g. projective identification) have also ceased. Intrapsychically, however, the search for an object does not seem to have been completely extinguished, perhaps also because the mother kept activating hopes in the boundary stretches.

I.e. we have the following initial situation: early traumatic events encountering a non-psychicised ego; encapsulation of these traumas; failure of objectal projection and withdrawal of interpsychic communication; deposition of the encapsulation in non-psychicised body; reinforcement of the arousals around the encapsulation by the sexually experienced boundary stretches; development of autistoid defence measures.

The dynamics can be derived from these psychogenetic, structural components.

The encapsulated contents can be felt by those who are affected as a dull throbbing deep inside the body. However, they are not felt as belonging to the self, but as alien, uncanny, threatening, exhausting. If these capsule contents are released, for whatever reason, the self is almost immediately threatened with unintegration.

Threatened with dissolution, the residual objectal hopes are called upon: Sometimes the sufferers still turn to (external) objects, but since the projective identification is no longer intact, they encounter no receptive object. The dynamic is shifted into the intrapsychic and, despite fears of dissolution as a result of unintegrated release, takes on accelerated regressive dynamics in which rapid intrapsychic projective and introjective processes take place (see above all Rosenfeld 1958, 1964, 2004). Inner objects are invoked, which are only experienced in a denying or absent way. They do not alleviate. Thus the dissolution accelerates. The situation seems insoluble: The inner object (introject) does not contain; yet without an object, there is annihilation. The weakened self must find a solution: displacement of the traumatic elements into its most "valuable" organ, which is then offered to the introject (a fused super-ego).

To the introject the organ is presented on which existence hangs and which at the same time threatens it. This dynamic could be paraphrased as follows: "Here is my existence, but annihilation threatens, please let me be" – and with no hope in prospect, the self must then sense that there is only a shadow there, no sublation redeems. The elements have found a replacement capsule, but one that cannot exert any containing function; for the body has flattened out into the somatic region dominated by sensations, has lost its psychical shape (*Gestalt*) and the organ has degenerated into the autistic object. There is no development, only perseverance until the dynamic ebbs away.

IV Hypochondriac dynamic – a clinical example[19]

A highly intelligent patient comes from a family of intellectuals. For the patient the father was a complete failure, as an alcoholic. The mother used to campaign for the victims of persecution by dictatorships, virtually living for this involvement. In her social commitment she was unattainable for the patient, totally absorbed, "barricaded herself behind her victim crap." In one session he reports on an acute hypochondriac breakdown:

Patient: "I completely surpassed myself last week in the show [= theatre performance], incredibly; was proud and happy as anything. Superb, like a young god. The others were good too, great show. *(Quieter)* Thought, that'll reassure my parents. Didn't stay behind afterwards, though, to party with the others, got straight out of there instead, somehow."

Psychoanalyst: "You wanted to look for your mother?"

Patient: "Yes, I think so too, actually thought about ringing them, but didn't do it in the end, don't even know why, something stopped me. Then, still completely euphoric, went to a kiosk, which looked fairly crummy. So there was this woman, awful, grumpy face, not a word; she fished the Coke tin out of a grubby corner and pushed it across the counter, with a bored, hacked-off expression. Didn't give me a second look. Could already sense the euphoria fading as I slid downhill, then walked down to the subway. Panic, emotion, I'm coming apart, everything is disintegrating; didn't really see the cars, the houses properly any longer, spun around, went all dizzy. Then down at the subway I got angry; thought, that bitch; thought, if I was a dictator, I'd have her marched off, she'd grovel. Oh, what the hell: I'd have her pulverized. I was raging, drank the Coke, then saw that it was really grimy, with particles on top; fear, thought, rat poison or suchlike; I would have inhaled that poison, now my vocal cords are knackered, the poison will corrode them. Got out of there in a panic, vocal exercises, half the night, but the fear stayed with me."

The patient subsequently went to see various doctors. That fear, which also intensified into mortal fear of a brain tumour, persisted for a long time.

The patient appears proud, but despite his initially inflated mood, remains self-critical and object-related ("It'll reassure my parents"). But an affective, object-related idea, i.e. showing himself to his mother proudly, and she finally beaming at him now; and the hope of still establishing a good rapport with the parents nevertheless, adds virulence to traumatic experiences of an intrusive, simultaneously unattainable mother which he cannot process mentally; "somehow" he has to get "straight out of there." Relying on his own resources, he can no longer fix this mentally.

That is, object-libidinous hopes are still extant in the sublimation, even if a slight withdrawal into the self and into narcissistic delusions of grandeur may already be attestable as well. The hope of a receptive mother, however, is linked with trauma, which segues into the initial turmoil.

He needs an object that is able to receive in a loving-present way. Ever of good cheer, he consistently looks for his mother, who must be sensorily perceptible, however, since the incipient dynamics do not permit more mature modes (hence the idea of calling them). Since it again wrenches open the traumatic flank of an unattainable mother, this idea is inhibited ("didn't do it... something stopped me"). Yet the wish persists and is acted out by the ill-fated walk to the kiosk. He looks for his mother at the grotty kiosk and finds in the woman's attributes – awful, grumpy face, not a word, bored, hacked off, not looking – the non-resonant, non-containing mother. The failure of the external object is already an unconscious reiteration, a seeking-out of the traumatic.

The rejection experienced (vanishing of the euphoria) leads to the liberation of the encapsulated content and to the breakdown of the affective idea. These parts elude psychological access and threaten the psychical system. The threat allows initial depersonalised and derealised aspects to become visible (the patient no longer views the world properly). Once again, a two-sided projection should save the day: The internal objects, the kiosk woman and the dismissive yet needed mother are supposed to bear these poisonous nuclei within themselves, sense destructive fright and terror in the threat, feel what it is like to beg to be heard, to whine, to plead for mercy and humanity; that is, endopsychic-projective evacuation and sadistic mastery are at work here. The patient puffs himself up into the great dictator (cf. the mother's commitment to persecutees of dictatorships). The raging becomes increasingly ecstatic. The unconscious premonition that the maternal object remains indomitable and unattainable, and will not detoxify, no doubt leads to further escalation: The object is pulverised, annihilated. The fear of dissolution is liberated. Only one path to salvation still remains: the final re-introjection, which is accomplished in concrete terms and perceived as almost ad hoc ego-dystonic.

Here we can see the disintegrative processes that initially lead provisionally to psychotic formations (incl. megalomaniacal approaches) (see Freud and H. Rosenfeld). They are to be understood as a defence against the break-up, but do accelerate the regressive decay that leads to fragmentation and concretism.

At the instant of pulverised annihilation, the entropic capsule contents are finally released, the disintegrative dynamic is joined by an unintegrative one. The patient makes a poor attempt at a further rescue, in which the excessive excitations and autistoid measures come into play. In the patient's experience, the two-dimensional maternal object fuses with the primitive super-ego aspects. This "shadow" seizes possession of the particles and, taking cold revenge, divested of the dimensions that endow meaning and affiliation, forces them back into the patient. That is to say, it not only does not detoxify, but also deprives the kernel of what is probably its last psychical, objectal quality. This super-ego (Bion) itself becomes dictatorial, destructively menacing, and thus wrests from the self that megalomaniacal part, which loses its inflated size in the process.

The concretistic re-introjection of destructive particles of poison, which are inhaled and not imbibed, destabilises the patient's psychic system (recall here Fenichel's [1945/1982] observation, which pointed out that, in the case of hypochondria, the introjection takes place in a very bodily, oral, anal fashion, through the breathing or the skin, etc.). The patient's regressively weakened ego threatened with dissolution must do everything to avert the annihilation.

The shadow figure now makes possible restitutive measures. It permits the patient to offer up one of his most narcissistically cathected organs to the shadow for sacrifice – his vocal cords, in which he accommodates the toxic elements. Without functioning vocal cords the patient cannot take to the stage, and the phallic narcissism attached to sagacity, eloquence and musicality since his childhood collapses, i.e. the fixated method and hope for attracting the mother's attention. Consequently, the brain, that organ of sagacity, is also soon stricken by the tumour of no longer taming the fear.

The reasons for processing the hypochondriac crisis are grounded above all in the impossibility of transforming such released nameless states into psychic ones without a containing object. Hypochondria in its agitated form is an attempt to provide a last bulwark against an experience of dissolution that no longer appears "tangible," that is two-dimensional: submission to a "shadow," binding the extreme, perverse excitations in hypochondriacal agitation (orgiastic self-examinations, visits to the doctor, etc.) and abuse of the organ as an autistoid object. The fatal thing is that this dynamic no longer turns interpsychically to an object, but perpetuates the early child-hood lostness. The patients remain alone with the nameless states, as in their earliest childhood days. They have no capacity to discover this constellation within themselves. Therefore, according to my observations, treatments proceed similarly to the analysis of the breakdown described above.

2.4.2 The camouflaged nameless

I would like to describe an observation in which patients have a hyperrealistic perception that not only affects surfaces but extends to the inside of objects. I once called it "X-ray eyes for the innermost" (Nissen, 2021).

Stories as autistic objects are well known (see Barrows, 2001), also the insu-larity of people with autistic disorders to hyperrealistic and hyperexact percep-tion. In 2008 I described a man who told stories (observations of everyday events as well as things he had experienced himself) in a form in which the narrative dominated - of a linguistic brilliance and visual complexity that was so aston-ishing that speaker and listener almost vanished. They were hyperrealistic and hypersensual. For example, he described elderly women on the underground so precisely that one could see their shape, hear their noises and smell their smell. Yet it was striking that in a really unnarcissistic fashion he did not lie in wait for the reaction of the object. Telling stories was not interaction, not an interpersonal exchange. There was only the story-subject; object, speaker, listener did not exist. He also told himself such stories or lived in them. I understood these stories as an autistic barrier against internal and external reality. They do not serve com-munication, but act as an internal and external shield. In spite of the hyperreality, external impressions do not turn into mental perceptions, with internal impres-sions being hardly sensed, let alone turning into significant elements. The level-ling out to two-dimensionality and the reduction of time to only the present tense are becoming visible.

But this hyperrealistic and hypersensualistic mode can, I suspect, focus on an-other dimension, that of capturing internal states, dynamics, strivings, motives of objects so precisely that it seems like an unfolding and representation of the conscious, preconscious and unconscious world. But none of this is psychic. It is the perception of inner states and outer constellations that serves one's physical survival. This survival strategy has become independent and detached from threatening situations – and has taken the place of object relations. One could see similarities to the "as-if" personality (Deutsch, 1934), which undoubtedly also exists, but it is not really an assimilation to another, but a hyperexact registration of sensual states that is pretended as "understanding" of objects and relationships.

An example: A patient who grew up in the most difficult circumstances witnessed a violent quarrel between a mother and a two- to three-year-old girl, which took place in the neighbouring flat. I will try to capture her description, which made me experience the quarrel almost sensually:

> Uninhibited, the mother shouted, increasing without restraint, not knowing why, therefore becoming more and more violent. Her rage escalated into a will to destroy. Violence as intoxication, as feeling alive. She had gone too far, there was no turning back. The furor tolerated no admission. I knew the increase would soon need objects. And it came, something flew against the wall, a chair, a table, I don't know. I knew the little girl was standing there, frozen, not in fear or terror or anything, just frozen. Standing there was provocation for the mother. It was clear that the little girl had to get out of the mother's field of vision, not hide under the bed, that would be the next escalation, no, rather press herself into the corner of the window and look out motionless, afraid. Then the mother might have let off contemptuously. The little didn't make it. I rang the bell, otherwise it would have ended in physical violence.

The patient experienced traumatic-cumulative violence from her earliest days, in which she developed hyperrealistic observations as a survival strategy, in which she not only grasped the situation precisely, but learned to guess the inner strivings of the objects and was able to grasp her own states as if from a third perspective. This is probably how she was able to free herself from shock-like rigidity and paralysing fear as a child and develop responses to action that would ensure her survival. It may therefore be that this account of neighbourly violence is a realistic description of the situation. But there is no psychic quality here at all. Such reports were also never interpsychic messages; they were only indirectly addressed to me, namely, that the patient was giving me a chance to see something of these worlds. I felt that any reference to her person was not possible. If I did make genetic connections here, or tried to address her affects, she reacted by shaking her head in surprise – I then felt stupid and dull.

Some patients can also use this ability to grasp situations hyperrealistically to put themselves imaginarily into the lives of others, so that these worlds seem to them to be self-experienced. For example, a patient once said that he was familiar with the world of technical laboratories because his grandfather was the director of such a facility. It sounded like this, and I spontaneously believed him, that he had experienced these worlds as a grandson. But he had never met his grandfather.

The grandfather, who died early, already played no role whatsoever in his mother's family. Only the fact that there had been such a grandfather led into an illusionary, self-created world, which seems to be self-experienced through factual details.

How essentially nameless-dissolving this world of the patients is becomes apparent when their defences collapse. One patient reported that he was repeatedly subjected to "annihilation attacks"; he would then lie rigidly on the bathroom floor for "one or two days" (de facto 16–20 hours), letting himself go, motionless, annihilation panic, "every movement is the end, the dissolution" (quotation from patient) – a description that is somewhat reminiscent of Bion's stupor during non-existence. In another patient, sensory perceptions dissolve completely, a world emerges that seems even more disordered than primary-process thinking. I have described some moments of such dissolution elsewhere (see Levine (ed), 2022). The following quotation is reduced by me to a few sentences, much more confused in the situation, encompassing many minutes.

> I was with Max, suddenly he was standing in the room, we were wearing clothes, the child had, I had something with him once, sex, was it sex? 15 years ago, all full of rubbish. How did Ludwig get into the room? Crazy, huh? Sarah never came, not even in the evening. It was a party, really loud. There was nothing going on with Sarah, but she wants to give me her jacket. It's damaged, in the bin. W. (first name of an internationally known artist) was drunk, I've known him forever, with bottle. Sarah's in bed, at her party, can you imagine? Probably with Keith…

While the patient – much more confused and disoriented in the scene – is talking, she lies as if in shock, with a slight head tremor, while making defensive movements with one hand.

I will now first write what I knew about the material at this point:

Max is an older man with whom she fell a little in love. Ludwig was probably standing in the room where she was lying with Max, still dressed. Did Ludwig have a child in his arms? Ludwig is 75 years old, did she have sex with him 15 years ago? She wasn't even 10 years old then! Sarah, depressive acquaintance of her mother's age, probably had a party, was lying in bed (or is she still lying in bed?). Sarah once gave the patient a jacket, which she threw away, always afraid it would be discovered. The patient's father worked with W. at times. Keith's been dead for five years.

But I no longer had this knowledge at my disposal. For I was infected by the dissolution of thinking. A panic arose in me, I would go crazy, psychotic, if I continued to listen. This is not a paraphrase of a feeling or a countertransference, but a real fear, panic, from which I wanted to flee inwardly. I wanted to get out of my body, felt helpless, at the mercy, panicked that this was not possible. I know all kinds of reactions to similar material (depersonalising, distancing, e.g. taking refuge in rationalising, etc.). But in this scene the threateningness was different: a being at the mercy and a panic threat that it would really happen, happen unavoidable.

How can these observations be understood? It seems to me that these patients live in an unreal, hallucinatory parallel world. They connect with the psychic world of objects only through the hyperrealistic/-precise powers of observation with which they can camouflage themselves almost perfectly. Strictly speaking, however, this hyperrealistic experience is not a perception of independent sensations, but is ultimately a self-generated hallucinosis-like entity.[20] These productions are connected to the world through the traumatic life history and help to find one's way in the world. However, they are not the basis of sensuality from which psychic entities can emerge. The scanning of the world serves the adaptation and metamorphosis, at the same time the recognition of possible dangers. If the adaptation fails or the dangers break through the autistoid defences, it is felt, as in autism, as a tear in this hyperrealistic second skin, which lets what is held together fall apart and collapse and the dangerously foreign decompose everything. As long as the hyperrealistic façade remains closed, a subtle pressure is exerted on the objects (which often manifests itself in a diffuse unease) to act along, e.g. to deny the "Escher-like" with secret craziness (Krejci, 2012).[21]

2.5 The distressed ego – abandoned by all senses

Even though there are strong metapsychological, theoretical and clinical differences in the spectrum of "nameless states" (non-existence; breakdown; autistic/autistoid states; traumatisation; also somatoform/psychosomatic states), in my opinion three converging lines can be identified:

- The states are not psychicised or have not acquired sufficient psychical meaning. They are thus excluded from psychic intercourse; unconscious phantasies are largely absent.
- They are not objectal or have fallen out of the objectal dynamic; communication from Ucs to Ucs is disrupted, and projective identification fails.
- They persist actual, i.e. they are experienced as present, and, being exempt from psychic intercourse, are relatively resistant to change. They hardly process and differentiate.

If these three characteristics are true, I think there are some theoretical-clinical implications.

We have a difficult situation before us: There are non-psychicised states that have fallen out of objectal intercourse. We cannot directly address these states with the methods that psychoanalysis has developed for areas of the repressed unconscious (in the broadest sense) and which operate objectally. Technically, this means that transference interpretations and symbolic interpretations, even those of concretistic and psychotic dynamics, are not helpful, since these operate in the objectal and remain interpsychically perceptible.

But the problems lie not only in the realm of the object relation, but also in the fact that the raw elements and the untransformed β-elements have not acquired psychic meaning. Put simply, the ego/self has to deal with elements that are exempt from psychic processing; indeed, that can no longer even be expelled.

The resulting distress should not be underestimated. Once, the failure of unconscious communication and projective identification is perpetuated. It is experienced as a sensory-bodily tension that cannot be communicated. But, furthermore, this tension has another cause: The self/ego cannot take experimental cathexis (Probebesetzung); the elements are no good as signals.

To understand this, Freud's reflections on anxiety might be helpful. Freud's theories of anxiety have changed a lot: If the earliest models (in the beginnings of psychoanalysis) still seem to assume a physical-biological process, the theory of anxiety developed in the Interpretation of Dreams and in the metapsychological writings is quite complex, not reducible to the thesis that "unsatisfied libido was directly changed into anxiety" (1933a, 82). For in both "The Repression" and "The Unconscious," more complex models are outlined in which the "quantitative factor of the instinctual representative has three possible vicissitudes...: either the instinct is altogether suppressed, so that no trace of it is found, or it appears as an affect which is in some way or other qualitatively coloured, or it is changed into anxiety" (1915d, 153; see also 1900a). And in "The Unconscious" it says:

> Excitation ... must ... give rise to a slight development of anxiety; and this is now used as a signal to inhibit, by means of a fresh flight on the part of the cathexis, the further progress of the development of anxiety.
>
> (1915e, 183)

In the so-called second theory of anxiety, the ego is the actual seat of anxiety (1926d, 92): "... anxiety makes repression and not, as we used to think, the other way round, and ... the instinctual situation which is feared goes back ultimately to an external situation of danger" (1933a, 89). With this "neurotic anxiety has changed ... into realistic anxiety, into fear of particular external situations of danger" (1933a, 93).

The ego "makes use of an experimental cathexis [Probebesetzung] and starts up the pleasure-unpleasure automatism by means of a signal of anxiety" (1933a, 90).

But the basic situations of danger are different for nameless states:
The essential thing of such states is, that

> they call up in mental experience a state of highly tense excitation, which is felt as unpleasure and which one is not able to master by discharging it. Let us call a state of this kind, before which the efforts of the pleasure principle break down, a *traumatic* moment. Then, if we take in succession neurotic anxiety, realistic anxiety and the situation of danger, we arrive at this simple proposition: what is feared, what is the object of the anxiety, is invariably the emergence of a traumatic moment, which cannot be dealt with by the normal rules of the pleasure principle.
>
> (1933a, 93f)

So there is for Freud "no objection to there being a twofold origin of anxiety – one as a direct consequence of the traumatic moment and the other as a signal threatening a repetition of such a moment" (1933a, 94f).

Freud is operating here with a very broad concept of trauma, which is present when the pleasure-unpleasure principle fails. However, if we take his considerations from other writings into account, we can define the concept of trauma more narrowly: a state of absolute helplessness and of highly tense excitation that can no longer be managed by discharging. What we called encapsulation is thus a traumatic moment that singularly or cumulatively constitutes such a danger of dissolution that the ego can no longer take defensive measures via signals, but is in danger of being pulled into the abyss. I.e. the signals can no longer be used for anxiety regulation and interpsychic communication, but are indistinguishable from dissolving entropy.

If the ego chooses the perverted solution, it loses its most important functions, namely, many of the characteristics of system Cs. If it actively seeks the excitement that ultimately heads for dissolution and tries to redirect it into perverse pleasure, it not only removes itself from the object relations, but also loses functions of the reality principle and the secondary process. The barter is bad: What is "won" in this dynamic is the addictively perverse excitement, which is sometimes heightened to the orgiastic. But a malignant spiral develops: Reality has to be increasingly denied, the ego functions are withdrawn, the object is lost. A perverse-autistoid world develops in which an understanding object no longer appears.

The ego can now only secure its existence, or that of the self, with primitive measures, namely, mobilising autistoid defences in the narrower sense, which, first, can be self-generated and in which, second, many functions of the reflexive ego are switched off. Autistoid forms and objects, for example, can "lull" the self into a trance-like state; second skins create adhesive bonds next to which nothing seems to exist.[22] The constructive-objectal part of the self floats away into increasing isolation and lostness.

Technically, we must recognise this distress of the ego and understand perversion and autistic measures as emergency operations with which it wants to secure its existence, while at the same time increasing the dangers. Not only can the ego not take experimental cathexis and not use signals, it must avoid any approach to the nameless. However, it cannot avoid the excesses of perverse excitement and the adhesive two-dimensional flattenings, but a new problem immediately arises: These states have no psychic quality and elude revision. Here, too, the ego experiences itself as helpless, since it cannot bring about any change of its own accord. What is more, experimental cathexis and signals cannot be used, but threaten to tear into the abyss. The constructive ego may now under certain circumstances mobilise hope in an object. But the invocation of the object also fails: The ego is hardly able to communicate the experience of such perverse-autistoid states, so that the practitioner hears the words but, since they have no psychic meaning, cannot understand them. This non-understanding is usually perceived by the patients as very agonising. Thus, although we hear descriptions such as those in the case vignettes, e.g. of orgiastic, hypochondriacal self-examinations, experience coprophilic practices, listen to descriptions of depressive dying, they are usually not psychically connectable; indeed, sometimes it seems as if they cannot be grasped at all.

This phenomenon could perhaps be explained with the following speculation: *The elements not only have no psychic quality, but no differentiated sensual quality* (see Chapter 4.1), since excitation and damping, pleasure or pain dominate in the perverse-autistoid deformations. Differentiated sensual qualities are swallowed up by these dominant regulations. The sensual qualities thus do not "contain" the quantitative dimensions, but excitation and attenuation level sensual experience.[23] This view would make more understandable the clinical experience of practitioners who repeatedly describe that they are not even able to grasp the sensual level of experience. Thus it is almost universally the case that hypochondriacal complaints, in which patients speak stressfully of fear of death, leave us "completely cold." Even coprophilia, which always triggered aversive reactions in my colleagues, did not produce any resonance in me (until the touch of wet hands).

With such a view, the technical problems of treatment emerge ad hoc. In nameless states, the hope for an understanding/holding object is abandoned. And elements have not only not been sufficiently psychically qualified, but stripped of their sensual qualities. But if not only the objectal-psychic is disturbed, but even the sensual is reduced to a binary pleasure-unpleasure, and perhaps even this binary is no longer allowed to register, then statements by Freud and Bion on the reduction of the sensual to pleasure and unpleasure become more understandable and truly massive technical problems arise.

Notes

1 Grotstein distinguishes between "pre-conception" (with hyphen) and "preconception" (Grotstein, 2007, 63, 87, see Bion, 1962, 70). "Pre-conception" is the a priori, unthinkable core of the unconscious, which becomes noticeable in the mental area as an expectation. "Preconception," on the other hand, is an a posteriori, already saturated conception which becomes pre-knowledge and eventually leads to the acquisition of human reason. Besides this epistemological distinction between pre-conception, preconception and premonition, Bion (1963) discusses in detail the ambiguity of these expressions, e.g. in Chapters 16, 18, 19 of Elements of Psychoanalysis.
2 This is quite in line with Bion's view: The pre-conception "... is a state of mind adapted to receive a restricted range of phenomena" (1963, 23).
3 Wherever possible, for reasons of confidentiality, I try to make use of published case material, which is then discussed from new points of view (see Nissen, 2013).
4 Freud probably destroyed a work on consciousness in the context of his metapsychological investigations. It seems to me that it is difficult to interpret Freud's view (e.g. 1900a; 1911b; 1915 c, d, e; 1917d; 1920g; 1923b; 1940a) coherently: Perception – Pcpt system – Consciousness – System Consciousness (Cs) – Pcpt-Cs – Preconscious (Pcs) – Ego are not clearly separated. Freud sometimes equates perception and consciousness, but the Cs system does not seem to coincide with the Pcpt-Cs, etc. It is noticeable that Freud, e.g. in 1911b, repeatedly recurs to the ego (Ich) concept where he addresses the system Cs, but notices that it is topically interwoven with Pcs.
5 In "Learning from Experiences," Bion drops the distinction between inner and outer world (1962, Chapter 2, 1). Sense data of the self therefore means that the inner and outer sense impressions are registered by the consciousness of the self.

6 See Bions discussion of premonition: "The term "premonition," as I propose to use it, represents emotional states rather than ideational content, thus leaving the term "preconception" to represent the latter... The premonition can therefore be represented by (Anxiety (ξ)) where (ξ) is an unsaturated element...

   Analysis must be conducted so that the conditions for observing pre-monitions exist ... If premonitions cannot be experienced correct interpretation becomes difficult for the analyst to give and difficult for the analysand to grasp..." (1963, 76) However, he does not take up this discussion again, although it seems important to me for the relation between idea and emotion (see also 1963, Chapter 19).

7 Bion makes clear, "In psycho-analysis any O not common to analyst and analysand alike, and not available therefore for transformation by both, may be ignored as irrelevant to psycho-analysis. Any O not common to both is incapable of psycho-analytic investigation..." (1965, 48f) and continues: "the transformation of the patient must always be the O that is transformed when the analyst works to arrive at an interpretation" (1965, 49).

8 An example would be a couple where the man has developed a drinking problem. Both "know" it, but the knowledge remains in splitting (see Freud, 1927e; 1940c). Then the woman states (T→O) to her husband: "You have a drinking problem." At this moment, alcoholism is there as a psychic reality, and at the same time the couple has become a different one. This catastrophic change rearranges the elements and subjugates the couple, causing quite severe anxiety.

9 See Bion's comments on hallucination (1965, 136f); also Tustin, who speaks of "self-generated sensations" in autistic objects (Tustin, 1986, 27).

10 Freud paraphrases this process: "'... I am the breast.' Only later: 'I have it'..." (Freud, 1938b, 299).

11 Zeitzschel (2018, 2022) tries, among other things, to describe early experience with the help of infant observation, thereby also identifying moments of dissolution.

12 See also Nissen (2016; endnote 3).

13 For me, this experience was one of the most important clinical experiences and has changed my understanding of severe depression in a lasting way. Since then, I have also been very critical of the general thesis of some psychoanalytical theories that suicide is always a murder of the object.

14 Pierre Marty once said: "You build psychosomatics out of its womb and out of its dead" (quoted from M'Uzan, 2020).

15 I owe the reference to a "phase of happiness" in such treatments to U. Moser (personal communication).

16 D.G. and D. Power see the magnitude of the change brought about by such a moment as follows: "According to Vermote ... so powerful did Bion believe the experience of at-one-ment to be that he believed one or two moments of at-one-ment allowed an analysis to be terminable" (2023).

17 In the moment of presence time and space reveal themselves (s. Nissen, 2022). Gadamer writes: "Time is for being to happen" ("Zeit ist, dass Sein sich ereignet." 1969, 143). What being the philosopher Gadamer has in mind, I do not know, but I consider his determination of the time to be one of the most convincing.

18 By analogy with the damming-up of the object-libido in transference neuroses, Freud postulates a damming-up of the ego-libido in the case of paraphrenia and hypochondria, since the withdrawn "libido [...] does not remain attached to objects in phantasy, but withdraws on to the ego. Megalomania would accordingly correspond to the psychical mastering of this latter amount of libido, and would thus be the counterpart of the introversion on to phantasies that is found in the transference neuroses; a failure of this psychical function gives rise to the hypochondria of paraphrenia" (1914c, 151).

19 See Nissen (2000, 2018).

20 The question of whether these self-generated states could be a subtype of hallucinosis (see Chapter 3.2) should be investigated, as should the question of how these states relate to the nameless.

21 Krejci (2012) describes private/secret madness as the analyst's attempts at repair, in which he "sensibly" transforms meaningless, broken, faulty messages from the patient. The therapist operates – to protect his own self – with an adhesive, cuddly, autistoid defence. A fatal counter-acting out (enactment).

22 A small self-experiment can give an idea of such states: If we try to meditatively switch off all reflexive thinking and then mechanically, rhythmically press a spinning top for minutes – then a world-distant, trance-like condition arises that protects against everything dangerous, and in the nameless this is the real and psychic reality.

23 This process seems similar to that observed by Bion in stammering: "The words that should have represented the meaning the man wanted to express were fragmented by the emotional forces to which he wished to give only verbal expression; the verbal formulation could not 'contain' his emotions, which broke through and dispersed it as enemy forces might break through the forces that strove to contain them" (1970, 94).

Chapter 3

Methodical and technical issues

3.1 Free-floating attention and free association

Free-floating attention and free association are methodical and methodological concepts rarely mentioned by Freud, but in my opinion they are the fundamental methods of psychoanalysis. All other instruments of treatment are subordinate to these.[1]

First of all, we must realise that both principles are revolutionary discoveries: Free association[2] is a completely new text form (i.e. no description, no report, no argumentation, no logical deduction, no narrative, no speech, etc.). For them, narrative constraints that dominate normal communication do not apply, such as the constraints of gestalt closure, condensation and detail (Gestaltschließungs-, Kondensierungs-und Detaillierungszwang), i.e. a narrative must have a closed gestalt, be sufficiently detailed and condensed so as not to cause interactional interference (see Schütze, 1982). In the same way, free-floating attention runs counter to all polite and normal communicative habits, complementary duties of listening are suspended, the receptive attitude dims down to such an extent that natural protest against the free-associated disorder is absent.

Free-floating attention is the necessary counterpart to the demand made on the patient that he should communicate everything that occurs to him (1912e, 112). Freud goes on to write, with dry masterliness: "He should withhold all conscious influences from his capacity to attend, and give himself over completely to his 'unconscious memory.'" Or, to put it purely in terms of technique: "He should simply listen, and not bother about whether he is keeping anything in mind." Therefore, no strained attention, no intentional noticing, but an artificial fading out (Freud in a letter to Andreas-Salomé, 1916; 1980, 327). We must keep everything similarly suspended in free-floating attention while also allowing our intuition to work.

The patient's freely associated communications are searched in a free-floating way, to identify his unconscious.

Freud writes:

> Just as the patient must relate everything that his self-observation can detect, and keep back all the logical and affective objections that seek to induce him to make a selection from among them, so the doctor must put himself in a position

DOI: 10.4324/9781003434207-4

to make use of everything he is told for the purposes of interpretation and of recognizing the concealed unconscious material without substituting a censorship of his own for the selection that the patient has forgone. To put it in a formula: he must turn his own unconscious like a receptive organ towards the transmitting unconscious of the patient ... so the doctor's unconscious is able, from the derivatives of the unconscious which are communicated to him, to reconstruct that unconscious, which has determined the patient's free associations.

(1912e, 115–116)

So free association is the requirement to communicate everything that is caught by self-observation, without any regard to secondary-process objections. It is about developing an attitude that allows association to occur autonomously: "it" should speak from the patient – or more precisely: "It" should express itself.

The "necessary counterpart" is free-floating attention. One does not work without the other. For this also the analyst must adopt a position, therefore take an attitude in which "it" listens in the analyst – or more precisely – "It" registers in us.

Freud comes very close to what Heimann later developed in her work on countertransference when he writes that "everyone possesses in his own unconscious an instrument with which he can interpret the utterances of the unconscious in other people" (1913i, 320). Elsewhere it says: "It is a very remarkable thing that the Ucs. of one human being can react upon that of another, without passing through the Cs" (1915e, 194).

This more descriptive version could be understood methodologically and theoretically/metapsychologically as follows:

Freud conceives the psychic apparatus in the Interpretation of Dreams in such a way

that this apparatus, compounded of ψ-systems, has a sense or direction. All our psychical activity starts from stimuli (whether internal or external) and ends in innervations. Accordingly, we shall ascribe a sensory and a motor end to the apparatus. At the sensory end there lies a system which receives perceptions; at the motor end there lies another, which opens the gateway to motor activity. Psychical processes advance in general from the perceptual end to the motor end.

(1900a, 537)

This simple model is then extended by "memory-traces," which are connected according to the laws of association (simultaneity of occurrence, relations of similarity, and so on) and can take over memory function. The Pcpt system has no memory, but can grasp the whole variety of sensuality. Freud now adds to his scheme the psychic systems Ucs and Pcs (Figure 3, 1900a, 541), finally consciousness as sense organ directed towards that external world. The absence of the hallucinatory wish fulfilment forced a

new principle of mental functioning ... what was presented in the mind was no longer what was agreeable but what was real, even if it happened to be disagreeable. This setting-up of the *reality principle* proved to be a momentous step.

(1911b, 219; see also 1917d)

In this, attention was a function "which had periodically to search the external world, in order that its data might be familiar already if an urgent internal need should arise" (1911b, 220). The systems Ucs, Pcs and Cs are separated by censorships.[3]

The dream must come to terms with these realities. Freud writes: "the state of sleep makes the formation of dreams possible because it reduces the power of the endopsychic censorship" (1900a, 526). But reduce does not mean sublated. The censorships remain intact, so that the dream must evade them (1900a, 526 & 574). Thus, there is a progredient and regredient movement:

> The first portion was a progressive one, leading from the unconscious scenes or phantasies to the preconscious; the second portion led from the frontier of the censorship back again to perceptions. But when the content of the dream-process has become perceptual, by that fact it has, as it were, found a way of evading the obstacle put in its way by the censorship and the state of sleep in the Pcs.
>
> (1900a, 574)

In his metapsychological reflections on the dream, Freud argues that the narcis-sistic sleep state can be disturbed by internal as well as external stimuli. The re-pressed, as well as day's residue, has escaped the general withdrawal of cathexis. With such a cathected idea, "the preconscious dream-wish is formed, which gives expression *to the unconscious impulse in the material of the preconscious day's residues*" (Freud, 1917d, 226). The resistances (censorships) and the absence of motor discharge in sleep lead to the fact that "the content of the presentation not being thought, but transformed into sensuous images, which one then believes and thinks one is experiencing" ("daß der Vorstellungsinhalt nicht gedacht, sondern in sinnliche Bilder verwandelt wird, denen man dann Glauben schenkt und die man zu erleben meint" (1900a, G.W. 540; S.E. 535; Translation BN)). This is not easy to understand, since the Pcpt system is at the sensitive end, but is now innervated by ideas.[4] Why is it otherwise in dreams?

> The only way in which we can describe what happens in hallucinatory dreams is by saying that the excitation moves in a retrogressive direction. Instead of being transmitted towards the motor end of the apparatus it moves towards the sensory end and finally reaches the perceptual system. If we describe as *progressive* [progredient BN] the direction taken by psychical processes arising from the unconscious during waking life, then we may speak of dreams as having a *regressive* [regredient BN] character.
>
> (1900a, 542)

That is a "reverse direction, starting from thoughts, to the pitch of complete sensory vividness" (1900a, 543). Freud further remarks, "that it is not only in dreams that such transformations of ideas into sensory images occur: they are also found in hal-lucinations and visions" (1900a, 535).[5] In another place it says: "The formation of the wishful phantasy and its regression to hallucination are the most essential parts of the dream-work, but they do not belong exclusively to dreams" (Freud, 1917d, 229).

Freud also made the observation that "if memories become conscious once more, they exhibit no sensory quality or a very slight one in comparison with perceptions" (1900a, 540). The reverse direction, i.e. from presentation to perception, now makes it possible for the presentation to be "sensualised," i.e. to find a figuration independent of real sensory perception.

If we transfer this model, to which Botella also refers in a different form, to the interlocking methods of free-floating attention and free association, these can be taken out of the descriptive version and become theoretically more comprehensible.

3.1.1   Free-floating attention and free association in repression

Let us first stay with repressed states. Free-floating attention and free association represent attitudes that are entered into and adopted in the analytic process. They mean above all a disciplined lowering of the reality principle and secondary process. There are two consequences for the mental apparatus: (1) Objections of the reality principle and secondary process recede, control and selection of thoughts are reduced. The censorship between Cs and Pcs loosens. (2) The defence at the first censorship between Pcs and Ucs becomes more permeable; descendants can rise more and more undisturbed.

But the resistances are, not unlike the dream, only reduced, not eliminated. In free-floating attention and free association, descendants show up more easily and more disorderly (as the dynamic approaches the primary process). They show, as Freud observed, little sensual and psychic quality,[6] but nevertheless push towards representation (Darstellung). Similar to dreams, a regredient process can now unfold more easily in free-floating attention and free association, making the presentations sensually alive.[7] The presumed unconscious connection between patient and analyst can make it easier to find suitable representations (Darstellungen). This means that when important functions of the Cs system are reduced, the reverse direction can occur and the Pcpt system (Pcpt-Cs) can take effect, so that associations (presentations) become sensual.

If we now fall back on the theory of pre-conceptions, these elements (sensual presentations) can be connected into the preconceptual (without hyphen) structure and begin to allow a *psychic* complex, which (according to Freud) has conflictual potential, to emerge. This complex can be registered, ordered and constellated (Bion) by the free-floating attention, finally grasped as a conscious presentation. Thus, it can be brought into the relationship and a realisation can occur. As already explained, realisation is only possible in the relationship (if it remained as a conscious presentation in the analyst, it would be a process "in effigie" in which, as Freud wrote, one cannot slay the conflict).

A small example can illustrate this dynamic.

A patient of mine came to treatment, among other things, because of violent impulse outbursts towards his wife (he called such days "black days") and infantile-persistent conflicts with his parents. After we had talked for many months about his defended love for his mother, he "suddenly" shared a scene of his childhood in a density (in the present tense) that cannot be reproduced in words – how he went to fetch milk in the spring sun breaking through the tender greenery, holding his mother's hand, who was wearing a cream-coloured dress that billowed slightly in the wind. Everything was present: the beautiful mother, the tender touch of her, the suffusion of love and happiness, the light, the colours, the sun, the wind, the milk.

His "ability to love" was palpable before this association, his love for his mother undoubtedly existent. But they were warded off. This fact is very important. Through the loosened censorship between Cs and Pcs, the defences and resistances that do their work along the censorship between Pcs and Ucs become palpable. With Freud: The thing presentations (love of the mother/love of the woman) can be sensed, but the connection to the word presentations is missing. Since violent conflicts are at work, it should not become recognisable which love it is, it should not show itself psychically qualified and conceptualised. But the mill of the interlocking method of association and attention is slow, but it grinds. Thus, in a free association, the patient finally is able to let this love be there sensually in a very intense, "painted" scene.

I.e. the love for the mother (in its individual, psychic quality) was subject to defence, was, since the censorship between Cs and Pcs had become permeable, clearly felt as resistance in the transference. Part of the unconscious conflict finds its way progredientily into a screen-memory (fetching milk from the mother's hand). In the scene, the conflictual presentation "love for mother" is now transformed into sensual images in a regredient process. This pre-conception, having become sensually accessible, can thus become in the transference and be grasped and interpreted definitionally as a psychic presentation, i.e. word and thing presentation combined. The "realised" love revealed the oral and Oedipal desires quite undisguisedly: the almost paradisiacal, tender oral world in being breastfed (milk) and the Oedipal happiness of being exclusively at the mother's hand, making the father outside this exclusivity as if non-existent. This conception of "love for the mother" can be used further on to understand the missing, conflictual parts of the complex. For example, this love may have been inhibited with the threat of castration or may have turned into grievance and anger through a severe disappointment. In this patient, a severe disappointment related to the realisation of the exclusionary sexual relationship of the parents could be discovered as the cause of his "black days."

It becomes clear that a repressed complex can nevertheless be sensed in the defence; that the interaction of free association and free-floating attention finally generates a screen-memory that emerges as a presentation in a progredient and is sensually imaged in a regredient way; that psychic qualities and conceptions thus emerge and become in the relationship. I.e. the sensual is necessary alongside the (pre)conceptual dimensions for understanding the repressed complexes.

Freud, to my knowledge, did not explore the clinical-theoretical implications that arise almost inevitably and naturally from this derivation. In my opinion, the progredient and regredient dynamics, the "sensualisations," the more freely flowing transitions between the systems, etc., force us to adopt attitudes and methods that today are known as "dreaming." Artificial fading, free association and free-floating attention (which includes reverie) are inconceivable without dreaming and sensualising. Freud, on the other hand, directed his attention to clinical phenomena, which in the basic methods particularly allowed conclusions to be drawn about unconscious complexes.

I will briefly touch on these as they are relevant to my reflections on the treatment of nameless states.

Since, as we have already heard, psychoanalysis historically focused its investigations on the repressed, all avenues that contributed to the decoding of this sub-area of the unconscious were relevant. I can only present a minimal, arbitrary selection.

The concept of resistance, to which we already attributed great influence in the last chapter, runs through the whole of Freud's work. If it is still grasped in the beginnings as an obstacle to be overcome (e.g. in the "Studies" (1895d)), it is soon recognised as a means of gaining access to the repressed. The forces that have caused the repression, together with the attraction of the libido by unconscious complexes, will raise resistance to the analytic work (see treatment writings, e.g. 1912b). Soon, however, the resistance is attributed to the ego (see 1920g, 17f; 1933a, 158f), which "treats recovery itself as a new danger" (1937c, 238). It goes on to say, "The ego ceases to support our efforts at uncovering the id; it opposes them, disobeys the fundamental rule of analysis, and allows no further derivatives of the repressed to emerge" (1937c, 239).

When the patient commits to the fundamental rule, the resistances show up in many forms, e.g. disregarding the fundamental rule, specific breaks in association, failure to come up with ideas, flattening of the material, etc. They can be traced as nodes by the free-floating attention. Free association is one of the most effective methods of making resistance visible, thus tracking down repressed material. Resistance, in this view, is a phenomenon of the transference relationship, is thus involved in psychic and objectal dynamics.

The same applies to the transference: The patient transfers hostile as well as loving, including friendly tender and sexual feelings to the analyst, so that the conflicts that led to the neurosis are revived in the relationship with the analyst. This situation, which at first appears to be difficult, in reality offers us our great opportunity.

> Instead of having to deal as best we may with conflicts of the remote past, which are concerned with dead circumstances and mummified personalities, and whose outcome is already determined, we find ourselves involved in an actual and immediate situation, in which we and the patient are the principal characters and the development of which is to some extent at least under our control.
>
> (Strachey, 1934, 132)

Similar to resistance, Freud discovered that the transference can become a powerful weapon. The resolving of the transference neurosis succeeds with the transference – and with it the infantile neurosis.

Transference, then, is related to the central repressed contents and arises especially when these might be revealed. Freud's advice is: *"So long as the patient's communications and ideas run on without any obstruction, the theme of transference should be left untouched.* One must wait until the *transference*, which is the most delicate of all procedures, *has become a resistance"* (1913c, 139; second italics BN).

The scope of this sentence is immense. In order to slay the enemy, neurosis (Freud, 1912b, 374), it must be present. It becomes present through and in the transference. Then the advice to wait until it becomes a transference-resistance. When does the transference become resistance? In my opinion, when it becomes so violent that the presentation that had to be repressed forces its way into the relationship *in statu nascendi* and threatens to unfold *in vivo*. Then the conviction arises in the patient that the transference object (analyst) *becomes* the feared or beloved object of the conflict. Here we can see a direct line to Bion's "becoming."

M. Klein considered the transference as the central field on which the treatment takes place and is decided. She understands the transference as a total situation. According to Klein, all emotions, defence mechanisms and object relations of the self with inner and outer objects are transferred as a whole (Klein, 1952), as elaborated in detail by S. Issacs (1948) via the concept of unconscious phantasy. For Klein, this entire inner world is permanently transferred to the analyst, i.e. in the here and now, both the unconscious phantasies and the way they are enacted are permanently virulent and to be interpreted. Thus the interpretation of the transference takes on the most central significance.

Freud, however, did not only see the concept of transference, which he understood since the "Studies on Hysteria" (1895d) as the substitution of "some earlier person by the person of the physician" (1905e, 116), as a phenomenon between analyst and analysand, but also recognised its intrapsychic significance. Thus, it is said in the Interpretation of Dreams:

> We learn from the latter that an unconscious idea is as such quite incapable of entering the preconscious and that it can only exercise any effect there by establishing a connection with an idea which already belongs to the preconscious, by transferring its intensity on to it and by getting itself "covered" by it. Here we have the fact of *transference*, which provides an explanation of so many striking phenomena in the mental life of neurotics.
>
> (1900a, 562; italics in German original)

This transference of unconscious content to other areas is then also connected with repetition and acting out.[8]

He writes:

> …we may say that the patient does not *remember* anything of what he has forgotten and repressed, but *acts* it out. He reproduces it not as a memory but as an action; he *repeats* it, without, of course, knowing that he is repeating it.
>
> (1914g, 150)

Freud provides a crucial clue to why acting out should not (only) be deemed as negative:

> There is one special class of experiences of the utmost importance for which no memory can as a rule be recovered. These are experiences which occurred in very early childhood and were not understood at the time but which were *subsequently* [nachträglich – BN] understood and interpreted.
>
> (1914g, 149)

This means that acting out in the transference is an indispensable source of information, because the

> patient cannot remember the whole of what is repressed in him, and what he cannot remember may be precisely the essential part of it... He is obliged to *repeat* the repressed material as a contemporary experience instead of, as the physician would prefer to see, *remembering* it as something belonging to the past.
>
> (1920g, 18)

This present experience constitutes the high actuality and represents the field on which the victory must be won (Freud 1912b).[9]

Freud then brings together transference, acting out and repetition compulsion:

> The main instrument, however, for curbing the patient's compulsion to repeat and for turning it into a motive for remembering lies in the handling of the transference. We render the compulsion harmless, and indeed useful, by giving it the right to assert itself in a definite field. We admit it into the transference as a playground in which it is allowed to expand in almost complete freedom and in which it is expected to display to us everything in the way of pathogenic instincts that is hidden in the patient's mind. Provided only that the patient shows compliance enough to respect the necessary conditions of the analysis, we regularly succeed in giving all the symptoms of the illness a new transference meaning[1] and in replacing his ordinary neurosis by a "transference-neurosis" of which he can be cured by the therapeutic work.
>
> (1914g, 154)

Countertransference was soon recognised as an indispensable source of information. One can view Freud as understanding countertransference as a ubiquitous phenomenon, when he assumed that one's own unconscious was an instrument capable of interpreting the expressions of another unconscious (see above, 1913i). However, he also conceived of countertransference more narrowly and as an obstructive phenomenon which "arises in him [physician] as a result of the patient's influence on his ([physician] unconscious feelings, and we are almost inclined to insist that he shall recognize this counter-transference in himself and overcome it" (1910d, 144–145). Heimann expanded the concept (but see also the frequently overlooked work of Deutsch, 1926): "… the analyst's counter-transference is not only part and parcel of the analytic relationship, but it is the patient's creation, it is part of the patient's personality" (Heimann, 1950, 83). What is *indicated* in the word "creation" is that psychoanalysis is not only a process of revelation and discovery but also a creative one that takes place in the relationship.

It needs no further explanation that the clinical phenomena such as resistance, transference, transference-resistance, acting out, repetition and repetition compulsion, countertransference and the later precise investigations of enactments (see e.g. Feldman, 1999, 2007) have been researched primarily within the framework of repressed contents and are to be understood as psychic, thus objectal dynamics that are fundamentally different from nameless ones.

What is important for my argument, however, is that these concepts, which emerged from clinical phenomena, deepened and broadened the central methodology. Unlike Lacan, Laplanche & Pontalis, for example, who consider that the fundamental rule "contributes to the establishment of the intersubjective relationship between analyst and analysand as a *linguistic relation*" (Laplanche & Pontalis, 1972, 179; italics BN), I see free association as the *totality of the patient's expressed communications*. It is not possible not to attribute forms of non verbal expression, acting out, repeating, word choice, ideas, acoustic phenomena, etc., to the patient's communications (see also the work of Scharff, 2014, on these phenomena). Everything belongs to the patient's associations – and the analyst has to notice this totality free-floating.

A brief example to illustrate the complexity of this dynamic:

A patient says with low modulation that a dream fragment comes to his mind: "A young woman is walking down a street. Don't know what that's about either…" A long, too quiet silence.

I hardly see a woman in colour, rather black and white, walking down a street. But the scene seems like a picture from a long time ago. I experience the silence attentively, too quietly, immediately as a resistance in which the defence of isolation becomes palpable.

"Yesterday I went to the urologist, prostate cancer screening. Everything was fine."

Through the resistance, I connect the incidence with the dream fragment. So the incidence could be day residue. I ask if he can think of anything to say about the dream.

"Nah." Pause. "The woman had brunette hair. So it wasn't my wife, she has blonde hair."

I immediately "see" in the dream image the brunette hair standing out brightly. Delayed, I remember that the patient once mentioned that his mother had brown hair. Suddenly I also sense the transference in the resistance, respectively the transference-resistance.

What might the intrapsychic dynamics look like? Let us speculate:

First to the dream: A drive impulse is transferred in sleep to a repressed Oedipal presentation that connects with the day's residues. Homoerotic phantasies could perhaps play a role in the day's residue, but they would be difficult to reconcile with the woman in the dream. Castration fears are more likely to be preserved in the day's residue: Doctor = Authority = Analyst = Father. But the castration fear remains at a harmless level ("everything is all right"). Via the law of similarity, prostate can now be connected with prostitute. The dream thought "prostitute" cannot be represented sensually[10]; it has to be modified. Prostitutes are also called "streetwalkers," a term that can be well represented visually: "A woman (girl) walks down the street."

In short, the repressed Oedipal sexual desire is linked to its male gender, finds its way to the day's residues. Castration fears do not disturb sleep. Via the term prostate sexual desire (prostitute) is approached.

These relationships are there ad hoc in the transference: The patient tries to break this connection (resistance; isolation). But this process, being too silent, is noticed, so I ask for ideas about the dream. "Of course" he can't think of anything, then brunette hair, with the telltale addition: not his wife, who has blonde hair. Perhaps without the addition of brunette hair, I would not have remembered his mother's brown hair.

Freud famously drew attention to the "not." So is it his wife after all? Or is it his mother who is not his wife, but in the Oedipal is his wife after all? This would make the noticeable transference-resistance more understandable, since in the equation doctor-father-analyst I am directly involved.

I hope it will become apparent that the grasping of an interpsychic (transference) dynamic is not successful if it is reduced to the linguistic. It needs all channels, especially in the case of nameless states. Further developments in recent decades have examined "dreaming" (in the broadest sense) in free-floating attention more closely.

3.2   Bion's technical and methodical/methodological extensions

Bion's reflections have given rise to a variety of techniques and methods: reverie, α-function, dreaming, intuition, evolution, hallucinosis, dream-work-α. Bion does not use the term regredience, but his conception of dream, dreaming and hallucination is based on Freud's metapsychological definition of the dream, in which regression plays a decisive role (see above).

All of these terms go back to Bion, but they are not defined in a way that separates them, also because Bion often feels that implicit definitions and those ex negativo are more appropriate for the subject matter. However, a shift in the dominance of the terms is striking: If reverie, α-function are of central importance in "Learning," they no longer appear in "Transformations" and "Attention and Interpretation," while intuition and hallucination only become of great importance from "Transformation" onwards. The term dream-work-α is one from "Cogitation," but there it is equated with the α-function or simply α.

This shift, which probably also contributes to the understanding of the "post-Bionian approaches," which almost all refer to the "late work," goes hand in hand with two developments, in my opinion:

1 Bion seems, according to my thesis, to detach himself from the Kantian tradition. Hinshelwood suspects that he has engaged with Bergson's views (see Bergson, 1927 [2013], Chapter 4; also term élan vital), which include a critique of Kant, namely:

> Bergson challenged Kant, saying Kant showed how reason itself is the impediment to knowing the thing-in-itself. The constraints from space and time are the impediments which reason uses; and Bergson described a means of dismantling the apparatus of time and space, so that intuition, without space-time limitations, allows a knowledge of the thing-in-itself. That process of coming to the "real" thing-in-itself is Bergson's use of the term "intuition."
> (Hinshelwood, 2018, 207)

My speculation goes beyond that. I suspect that Bion knew Heidegger, since Heidegger's critique of Kant corresponds with Bion's O. Heidegger accuses Kant not only of making the recognition of Being impossible with the pure forms of intuition (time and space) and categories, but that Kant ultimately remained trapped in Cartesian thinking, namely, in the position that the possibility of recognition is grounded in the subject. Thus, he cannot grasp Being (Sein) as Beings (Seiendes) in its unconcealment (Unverborgenheit, "aletheia") (Heidegger, 1927; see also Grotstein, 2004).

2 Bion's clinical and treatment conceptions have changed considerably since 1965/67. He increasingly develops doubts about the classical methods of interpretation (Freud & Klein) and about gaining psychoanalytic insights. It is no longer the uncovering of the repressed, the discovery of states, conflicts, etc., that is in the foreground, but the binocular, bidirectional processes and movements. It is necessary to pay attention to the transformations that take place in the analytic relationship. The general principle is this: "(i) that the patient is talking about something (O); (ii) that something, O, has impressed him and that he has transformed the impression by the process represented by Tp α, and (iii) that his representation Tp β is comprehensible" (Bion, 1965, 17). The analyst is now confronted with the following situation: "O (analyst), the patient's statements, have been transformed by me, my mental processes being represented by T (analyst) α, to form a view, T (analyst) β, from which I deduce that T (patient)" = e.g. the weekend break (1965,17). This dynamic becomes the subject of investigation for different types of transformations: While the transformations as "rigid motions" still corresponded most closely to the classical transference process, in the projective transformations phenomena were examined in which

β-elements played an important role and which took place in a completely different relational space: "… events far removed from any relationship to the analyst are actually regarded as aspects of the analyst's personality" (1965, 30). In these processes there is a blending of self and object. The invariants, i.e. the characteristics that remain stable over the transformations, are quite easily recognisable in rigid motions, but only guessable in projective transformations. Bion notes: "To make a step towards definition of this space we consider it to be a K 'space' and contrast it with K 'space' – the space in which what is normally regarded as classical analysis takes place and classical transference manifestations become 'sense-able'" (1965, 115). In the case of projective transformation and transformation in hallucinosis, the invariants are so difficult to discern that the process of transformation itself (Tα), i.e. the processes of transition, thus the "caesura" becomes the focus of consideration: "Investigate the caesura; not the analyst; not the analysand; not the unconscious; not the conscious; not sanity; not insanity. But the caesura…" (Bion, 1975, 49).

The Language of Achievement comes to the fore with the "Negative Capability, that is, when a man is capable of being in uncertainties, mysteries, doubts, without any irritable reaching after fact and reason" (Keats, in Bion 1970, 125).

Let's take a brief look at Bion's conceptualisations of the central terms and then offer some reflections on the postbionic currents.

Bion reserves the term reverie "for such content as is suffused with love or hate" and understands it "as a factor of the mother's alpha-function" (Bion, 1962, 36). He understands reverie as a source of supply of "the infant's needs for love and understanding" (1962, 36). Aguayo (2018) argues quite convincingly that maternal reverie can hardly be distinguished from Winnicott's (1956) "primary maternal preoccupation,"[11] a condition of the mother, in which she "gradually develops and becomes a state of heightened sensitivity," a condition which could be "compared with a withdrawn state…" (1956, 302).

"By α-function I mean that function by which sense impressions are transformed into elements capable of storage for use in dream and other thoughts" (1963, 4). In the beginning of life the mother has to act as α-function for the infant. Bion calls the transformed elements α-elements; if the function is disturbed the impressions experiencing remain unchanged, become β-elements.

> Failure of alpha-function means the patient cannot dream and therefore cannot sleep. As alpha-function makes the sense impressions of the emotional experience available for conscious and dream-thought the patient who cannot dream cannot go to sleep and cannot wake up.
>
> (Bion, 1962, 7)

The α-function is thus active in waking and sleeping and permanently transforms impressions into α-elements. The "alpha-function, by proliferating alpha-elements, is producing the contact-barrier, an entity that separates elements so that those on one side are, and form, the conscious and on the other side are, and form, the unconscious" (Bion, 1962, 54) and works in the Pcs/Cs and in the Ucs. This makes it possible – according to Bion – "that the conscious and the unconscious thus constantly produced together do function as if they were binocular therefore capable of correlation and self-regard" (1962, 54). It thus collides with Freud's concepts of primary and secondary process as well as that of censorship.

Dreaming also takes on a broader meaning: "In other words, the dream-work we know is only a small aspect of dreaming proper – dreaming proper being a continuous process belonging to the waking life and in action all through the waking hours..." (Bion, 1992 [1959], 38). This also includes the analytical session: "...but that the dream and the psycho-analyst's working material both share dream-like quality" (Bion, 1970, 71).

The α-function thus produces elements from raw, sensual sensations that can be used for dreaming. This dreaming takes place not only at night, but day and night. So a progressive line, from the raw sensual into the psychic. But does the α-function also act on presentations, "sensualising" them again, as Freud described it, even if this sensualisation is without any background of sensuous reality?

This brings us to the domain of hallucination. Hallucinations "are not representations: they are things-in-themselves born of intolerance of frustration and desire" (Bion, 1970, 18). Why are they not representations?

> Ordinarily, constellation, constant conjunction, and binding (by nomenation) are a prelude to exploration of meaning. In the domain of hallucinosis the mental event is transformed into a sense impression and sense impressions in this domain do not have meaning; they provide pleasure or pain. In this way the unsense-able mental phenomenon is transformed into a beta-element which can be evacuated and reintroduced so that the act yields, not a meaning, but pleasure or pain.
>
> (1970, 37)

Let's try an illustration in an example: Let's imagine we are lying in the grass in the sun, a bit dozy. Leaves of grass touch our skin on the arm; the physical sensation does not become conscious (a kind of dozing "wake-up stimulus," as Freud calls it). Regrediently, an image of insects arises unconsciously. Thus cathected, the presentation becomes conscious. We look at the arm, see the grass, continue dozing. The reality check has saved our relaxation.

Let us imagine the same situation, skin sensations, a regressed image of insects. Now the dozing person looks at his arm. In the hallucination he now sees insects and passes over reality testing. "With this turning away from reality, reality-testing is got rid of..." (Freud, 1917d, 233).

We have already seen that the hallucination is a self-generated state, produced by ejected sensual elements. The pathological thing, however, is not the regredient visualisation (Bion restricts himself to this form), but that the hallucinator considers this state to be real and always present. So far Bion follows Freud. Now, however,

Bion opens up the subject matter: The hallucination can be overlaid by other phenomena (Bion, 1970, 36) and – thus concealed – not only persist, but determine the life of a person.[12] "To appreciate hallucination the analyst must participate in the state of hallucinosis" (1970, 36), that is, "become at one with his patients' hallucinations" (1970, 36). The renunciation of memory and desire is indispensable:

> Receptiveness achieved by denudation of memory and desire (which is essential to the operation of "acts of faith") is essential to the operation of psycho-analysis and other scientific proceedings. It is essential for experiencing hallucination or the state of hallucinosis.
>
> (Bion, 1970, 35f)[13]

With this understanding, it now becomes more comprehensible that the concepts of intuition and evolution become strongly significant. We have already quoted the ex negativo definition, namely, Bion's use of the "term 'intuit' as a parallel in the psychoanalyst's domain to the physician's use of 'see', 'touch', 'smell', and 'hear'" (Bion, 1970, 7). An intuitive understanding of intuition emerges. But what is intuited? That which evolves in a treatment session. Bion understands evolution as follows:

> In any session, evolution takes place. Out of the darkness and formlessness something evolves. That evolution can bear a superficial resemblance to memory, but once it has been experienced, it can never be confounded with memory. It shares with dreams the quality of being wholly present or unaccountably and suddenly absent. This evolution is what the psychoanalyst must be ready to interpret.
>
> (Bion, 1992, 381)

It goes on to say:

> This I have tried to do by speaking of one as "evolution", by which I mean the experience where some idea or pictorial impression floats into the mind unbidden and as a whole. From this I wish to distinguish ideas that present themselves in response to a deliberate and conscious attempt at recall; for this last I reserve the term "memory". "Memory" I keep for experience related predominantly to sensuous impressions: "evolution" I regard as based on experience that has no sensuous background but is expressed in terms that are derived from the language of sensuous experience.
>
> (1992, 383)

Elsewhere, Bion refers to Freud's letter to Lou Andreas-Salomé, 25 May 1916, thus himself associating intuition and evolution with free-floating attention (1992, 384). Bion himself then links intuition and hallucination:

> The proper state for intuiting psycho-analytical realizations ... can be compared with the states supposed to provide conditions for hallucinations. The hallucinated individual is apparently having sensuous experiences without any

background of sensuous reality. The psychoanalyst must be able to intuit psychic reality which has no known sensuous realization.

(Bion, 1967, 163)

Here the door is opened to a further understanding of hallucination: The psychic in itself is not sensual, so it must be grasped intuitively. One method can be the hallucinatory experience of the state that is being transformed. This hallucinatory experience must be clearly separated from dreaming (see below).

So much for a brief overview of Bion's important concepts. In my opinion, they can be fully integrated into the superordinate concept of free-floating attention: reverie as a part of primary maternity modified to the analysand, which represents a receptive posture in which regredient dreaming becomes easier. The α-function thereby acts on elements that are thus suitable for dreaming. Hallucinatory phenomena can emerge. A constellation then evolves from this floating that can be grasped intuitively. Intuition would thus be the ability to grasp the non-sensory psychic and let it become real in a moment of presence. With these attitudes, techniques and methods, within the framework of free-floating attention, states can also be approached that lie beyond the repression. They are therefore important additions. In my opinion, the fundamental change compared to Freud is the binocular interaction of the systems. So it is no longer: "Where id was, there ego shall be," but binocular digestion and working through in the systems, during the day as well as at night. This makes it ad hoc understandable that the "uncovering" of complexes is still necessary, but is only one step in the psychoanalytic cure.

3.3 Post-Bionian approaches

This is also where the post-Bionian approaches come in. Some works deepen and specify Bion's conceptualisations, while others focus on the non-repressed unconscious and seek answers to the challenges that arise from non-sensory comprehension.

3.3.1 Dreaming

Important studies were mainly concerned with dreaming.[14]

Ferro, who clearly defines the object of his investigations and the scope of his theory in scientific terms, even calls his method transformations in dreaming and narrative transformations.[15] He refers above all to Bion's reflections on "waking dream thought" and to the concept of the field, formulated by Baranger and Baranger (1961–62 [2008]). Psychoanalysis is less about content and memories, but about the development of capacities for dreaming, feeling and thinking. Ferro's "trick" is the following:

... the analyst precedes every communication by the patient with a kind of "magic filter" comprising the words. "I had a dream in which ..."; this represents the highest possible level of positive functioning of the field – namely, when the field itself dreams. Sense data are transformed by the α-function into thought.

(Ferro, 2009, 214)

With this magic filter, all associations are visualised almost naturally, including the non-psychicised parts:

By combining Bion's concept of waking dream thought with those of the field and of the characters of the session, we arrive at a space-time in which maelstroms of β-elements are transformed by the field's "α-function" into oneiric thoughts of the field.

(Ferro, 2009, 219)

Ferro (e.g. 2003, 2005, 2009) understands analyst and analysand as partners in a common field created by intertwined mutual projective identifications: "... the field is the locus that gathers together the projective identifications and histories of patient and analyst alike, who thus become co-protagonists" (Ferro, 2009, 217). "Unsaturated" interpretations process the shared dreaming that creates a unique narrative that enables transformations into the psychic. The material (associations, dreams, memories, sensual impressions, bodily sensations, etc.) thus acquires its own order, which the couple has created and which determines the couple. Mental illness depends on a defect in the transformation that occurs through α-function and dreaming; "it is only the expansion of the function of the whole dreaming apparatus that will lead us to healing." (Ferro, 2009a, 78; transl. BN)

However, this method is only applicable to patients who have sufficient α-function. Otherwise, the technique must be extended:

It goes without saying that all this applies to patients with a sufficiently well-functioning α-function (which generates pictograms). In the absence of this capacity to transform protoemotions and protosensoriality into pictograms (of the waking dream state), the analyst will need to cooperate, perhaps even using his own reveries, in the co-construction of the patient's α-sequences, thus enabling the patient to develop an α-function and containing capacity (♀) of his own and eventually allowing its stable introjection.

(Ferro, 2009, 218)

This is exactly where Ogden comes in. With an attitude of dreaming carried into the relationship, psychical processes can be released more easily. Ogden writes:

Many patients are unable to engage in waking-dreaming in the analytic setting in the form of free association or in any other form [...] "talking-as-dreaming" has served as a form of waking-dreaming in which such patients have been able to begin to dream formerly undreamable experience. Such talking is a loosely structured form of conversation between patient and analyst that is often marked by primary process thinking and apparent non sequiturs.

(Ogden, 2007, 575)

In this dreamy flow, de facto everything can be talked about, from daily events to "the taste of chocolate" (Ogden 2007, 575).

However, Ogden (2007, 575) insists that "the difference in roles of patient and analyst be a continuously felt presence." In the extension of this concept, active and formative interventions are also allowed. The aim of this broad version of dreams is to release the binocularly operating organs "conscious" and "unconscious" in the analytic process. However, this technique requires a lot of experience.

Ogden (1994, 98ff), however, does not see interpretations as sublated in "talking," but understands them as a becoming with recourse to Hegel's dialectic: since both the projecting and the recipient are partially and temporarily negated in their subjectivity, i.e. are ego and non-ego; they thus create a new subject:

> projektive identification can be understood only in terms of a mutually creating, negating, and preserving dialectic of subjects, each of whom allows himself to be "subjugated" by the other, that is, negated in such a way as to become, through the other, a third subject (the subject of projective identification).
>
> (Ogden, 1994, 100f.)

This intersubjective third then opens up new moments of understanding. In a later work, Ogden (2001; see also Ogden, 2004) extends this version and postulates

> that the dreams and reveries being generated by analyst and patient at the frontier of dreaming draw not only on the unconscious experience of analyst and analysand as individuals, but involve a set of unconscious experiences jointly, but asymmetrically, constructed by the analytic pair.
>
> (Ogden, 2001, 11)

One can understand this method in such a way that the analyst with his α-function helps the patient to dream states and elements that cannot be connected. In this way, states that cannot be processed intrapsychically undergo a transformation. Two aspects are important: The states become alphabetised, i.e. processible in the psychic apparatus – and this in the relationship that can be experienced holding and containing.

3.3.2   Hallucinosis

If these considerations differentiate methodical and methodological dimensions, many other postbionic works aim at the "psychic in itself," which is not sensuous, asking how to intuit psychic reality which has no known sensuous realisation.

Here the concept of hallucination/hallucinosis plays an increasingly important role, but is defined very broadly. Thus Civitarese postulates: "If he [Bion] speaks of hallucinosis it is because he wants to describe some scenarios touched by psychosis, in which there is no significant loss of contact with reality, and so no 'real' hallucination" (2015, 1092). Civitarese assumes that in this form of hallucination one can "wake up" at any time (2015, 1102). Hallucination is thus used almost congruently with dreaming.

In contrast, Miller (2023) describes a hallucination in which the important features of the hallucination are preserved in a very beautiful example: A schizophrenic patient reports a nightmare in which a train "pulverises" his head. Miller hallucinates a plate of spaghetti and tomato sauce. The hallucination only disappears when "something moves in me" and he becomes aware of it. In Miller's understanding, the analyst can thus replace the patient's missing hallucinatory ability, digest it for him; at the same time, the patient can experience an object that survives his nightmares. Miller does not interpret this event, but believes that it communicates itself through a kind of analytical primary maternity.

Here, then, we have a temporary "real" hallucination, which – according to my interpretation – is accompanied by an imminent collapse of the dreaming. In my opinion, this point is very important for understanding Bion's concept of hallucination and for distinguishing it from dreaming. A genuine hallucination occurs, which cannot be distinguished in principle from a psychotic one. Nor is it within the capacity, within the sovereignty of the hallucinating person to end this state. (I strongly disagree with Civitarese on both points.) In the hallucination something of the patient's psychic reality shows itself; it thus has *some* characteristics of a transformation in O (see also Miller description, who, e.g., feels no fear, nothing uncanny). This state would not be experienced in this way if the hallucinating person could "wake up at any time." The hallucination shows something of the patient's psychic reality unconcealed – and this event conceals itself again (see Miller: "something moves in me"). It has characteristics of a catastrophic change, i.e. it can lead to understanding or to a psychical crisis. Such processes represent a risk that cannot be averted by knowledge (K). Therefore, these processes go hand in hand with Faith!

In my opinion, however, it is not a transformation in O, even if Miller assumes a benign process via primary maternity. A transformation into hallucinosis is not a transformation in O. For this to happen, this experience would have had to become in the relationship. What is the O of the patient? It does not become clear because the interpretation is missing. I suspect that the O is not only the pulverised head, that is, the pulverised psychic thinking, but that this state is "always" there. The nightmare is a first attempt to "think" this state. But alone the patient (a human being) cannot do it; it has to become in the relationship. The presence moment includes the self, the object and the relationship. In the sublation of the presence moment, the nightmare, that is, the pulverised psychic existence, could find its first limitation, its first conception. The hallucinatory experience must be used to try to initiate a presence moment with an interpretation. Such an interpretation could be "A terrible image, it seems to me that you always live in such states…"

3.3.3 Intuition

The grasping of psychic reality, which many equate with O, also entailed further reflections on intuition. Bergstein encircles this concept with his reflections on caesura:

> The analyst's dreaming and intuition, perhaps a remnant of intra-uterine life, is elaborated as means of penetrating and transcending the caesura, thus facilitating

patient and analyst to bear unbearable states of mind and the painful awareness of the unknowability of the emotional experience.

(Bergstein, 2013, 621)

In his work, he arrives at an important definition of intuition:

Intuition is an unmediated knowledge or understanding of truth, not supported by any information derived from a familiar sensual source. Since it cannot be communicated to an other and cannot be corroborated by a rational method of scientific knowledge, it is often seen as close to mystical revelation.

(Bergstein, 2013, 623; see also Levine, who associates intuition with construction [2022, 40ff])

Vermote (2013; 2022) develops a three-zone model based on Matte-Blanco: Reasoning, Transformation in K and Transformation in O.

The first zone is the zone of Reason. This is finite, conscious verbal thought – perfect for operational problem solving...

The second zone is the zone of Transformation in Knowledge. Transformation in knowledge is a mixed finite/infinite functioning that is 95% unconscious... Representations originate here and govern us. Symbolizing, mentalizing, phantasy, creativity, dreaming and dream thoughts all originate in this zone of effortless psychic functioning... The last two decades, most psychopathology is explained in terms of the functioning/dysfunction of T(K). When something does not get symbolized or mentalized it is seen as pathogenic. This is currently the main explanation of psychosis, trauma, psychosomatics, anorexia nervosa and so on.

The third zone is the zone of O and transformation in O. This zone is outside verbal thought and representations and hence infinite, undifferentiated. It is a zone without distinction between internal/external, self/other and body/mind. Nevertheless, we can conceive some a-sensuous empty patterns in this zone, to use an expression of Augustine: forms in potentio. They are not yet expressed in sensuous forms and therefore mute, in the dark so to speak. At the deep fully infinite level is a silent "Dasein", a wordless pure experience- where direct intuitive contact is possible.

(2022, 129f)[16]

With Bergstein and Vermote, intuition becomes an entity that enables direct access to psychic reality, to at-ome-ment, to the "formless infinite."[17] The object is then no longer the pathological unconscious (including the repressed and traumatic), but the "unrepressed unconscious."

A very interesting connection between premonition, preconception and intuition is made by Eekhoff, who discusses Bion's allusions to premonition in detail:

...premonition emerges as the attractor of attention. Premonition, as the forerunner and the outcome of intuition, happens in relationship. It is a two-person event. Intuition links premonition with a preconception to create a "hunch" or a feeling outside of language.

(Eekhoff, 2003)

As for Bion (1963), premonition and intuition also become an important technical instrument for Eekhoff: "Premonition, as sensual manifestation of relationship, links with intuition to create an illusion of knowing. This healthy illusion provides order and cohesion, enabling the patient and analyst to find a center of gravity and a floor for experience" (Eekhoff, 2023).

3.3.4 Truth

The concept of truth and reality inherent in this now moves more and more into the centre of considerations that can be intuited (the term dream-work-α is also used, apparently as a new collective term). The aforementioned terms, especially intuition, are no longer part of a method, but become a new methodology:

It proposes a new analytic methodology that supplants awareness from its central role in the analytic process and, in its place, instates the analyst's (largely unconscious) work of intuiting the (unconscious) psychic reality of the present moment by becoming at one with it.

(Ogden, 2015, 285)

The unconscious psychic reality is equated with truth.[18]

It is against this background that the many works that circle around the absolute, ultimate truth are to be understood. Grotstein (e.g. 2004, 2009), who brings together dream-work-α, α-function and dreaming in a "truth instinctual drive" (2004, 1081), writes: "the subject must dream the absolute truth about ultimate reality into digestible personal truth" (2004, 1089). Some years later it is said: "Absolute Truth about an infinite, cosmic, impersonal Ultimate Reality, O, into a tolerable, finite, and acceptable personal truth" (Grotstein, 2009, 746).

This shift is moving away from genuinely analytical subject matter towards more ontological, indeed more mystical questions. In the meantime, it has gone so far as to borrow from quantum physics (e.g. uncertainty principle; entanglement theory) and to call for a "quantum psychoanalysis":

The essential being and at-one-ment at the heart of these revolutionary contributions [of late Bion and Winnicott; BN] regarding the patient's primordial unknown and unknowable psychic reality summon to my mind the quantum mechanics revolution in 20th-century physics; for with this revolution, we move into a probabilistic, entangled realm of unity rather than division, of profound interconnectedness rather than separateness, that operates at deep, invisible levels.

(Eshel, 2017, 785)

For Blass these ideas go "beyond the limits of psychoanalysis" (Blass 2012, 1441; also 2011); for me they are beyond serious scientificity.

Notes

1 I am arguing privately that Freud knew Eichendorff's famous poem "Mondnacht"/"The Moonlit Night," in which the floating of the soul is painted too unsurpassably.
2 Busch writes: "Freud gave us a method, free association, to help us understand not only what is on our mind, but why that may be" (Busch, 2018, 572).
3 The terms "attention" and "association" used in the Interpretation of Dreams (1900a) and in the Formulations (1911b) are quite compatible with the use of the same in "free-floating attention" and "free association."
4 In the "Entwurf" (1895 [1950a]), which contains many reflections on dream theory, Freud argues that in the "psychic primary process" perceptions are not securely separated from presentations.
5 It is important, and often misquoted, that Freud writes: "The *interpretation* of dreams is the royal road to a knowledge of the unconscious activities of the mind" (1900a, 608; italics BN). I.e. it is not the transformations of the dream or the dream itself that are the via regia, but their interpretation!
6 See above Freud: Conscious memories exhibit no sensory quality. In "Repression" Freud argues in a similar way: "The quantitative factor proves decisive for this conflict: as soon as the basically obnoxious idea exceeds a certain degree of strength, the conflict becomes a real one, and it is precisely this activation that leads to repression" (1915d, 152).
7 In this dissected, linearised representation, this process appears more chronologically causal than it is likely to be in reality.
8 Acting out had, accelerated by the failed English translation of the German "Agieren" as "acting out" (see Laplanche & Pontalis, 1972; Sandler et al, 1973; see also Klüwers exact historical depiction, 1995), acquired a pejorative connotation, which was not construed by Freud in this way.
9 Not until the '60s of the last century was acting out and its potential rediscovered. Anna Freud interprets her father at the International Congress in 1967 as follows: "Acting out in the transference within these limitations (meaning: the analytic rules: BN) was recognized in earliest times as an indispensable addition to remembering" (Freud, 1968, 166). With this return to the more neutral version of the concept the informative and epistemological potential became the focus of attention (e.g. Sandler's concept of role responsiveness; Klüwer's active dialogue; the concept of enactment).
10 Consideration of representability requires that the material (here "prostitute") can be represented sensually (in the dream above all visually), here "streetwalker."
11 Winnicott probably felt that this was almost plagiarism:

It is important to me that Bion states (obscurely of course) what I have been trying to show for 2½ decades but against the terrific opposition of Melanie. Bion uses the word reverie to cover the idea that I have stated in the complex way that it deserves that the infant is ready to create something, and in 'good enough' mothering, the mother lets the baby know what is being created…. I don't mind being shown to be wrong, or criticized or banged about. But I have done some important work out of the sweat of my psycho-analytic brow (i.e. clinically) and I refuse to be scotomized.

(Winnicott, quoted after Aguayo, 2018, 798; see also Hinshelwood, 2018, 204)

12 Sandler has studied, among other things, hallucinosis, in which people structure every relationship according to the pattern up-down, and has shown how subtle these movements can be (see e.g. Sandler, 2005, 2009, 2018).

13 Bion asks elsewhere, "What 'rules' govern the transformation of O into a visual hallucination rather than an auditory hallucination, or vice versa?" (1965, 62). I cannot discover an answer. His attempts to find the answer by recourse to Klein's theory do not seem appropriate to me (see e.g. 1965, 133).

14 Busch writes: "… while Bion is most often referenced for introducing the term reverie, it was Breuer (1893) who first coined the term to describe the hysteric's hypnoid state. Breuer also used the term "waking dream" to describe this state, which has come into the Bionian psychoanalytic perspective on technique…" (Busch, 2018, 570)

15 A very good summary of Ferro's reflections can be found in his 2009 paper, to which I refer primarily.

16 I have never heard a case study where this third zone became visible….

17 I have my doubts here; I see several veils in the moment of presence: Psychic reality shows itself in a specific, even more individual form that is not accessible to the reflexive ego. It has to become in the relationship, whereby both participants find individual presentative symbols. A direct intuitive contact is for me impossible.

18 Levine, discussing Ogden's work, points out that Ogden equates truth with many dimensions: reality, psychic reality, unconscious psychic reality, O (and external reality [Ogden, 2015, 295] BN). He asks: "…Ogden … refers to 'multiple coexisting, discordant realities', all of which are true'… If there are 'multiple coexisting, discordant realities', are there also multiple coexisting, discordant truths?" (Levine, 2022, 68f).

Chapter 4

Basic and practical-technical issues

4.1 Sensuality: further considerations

I would like to return to Freud's reflections on dreams and Bion's extensions of dream theory and offer some practical and clinical reflections on how states and elements that cannot be dreamed can technically be dealt with in treatments. Various concepts have been developed; we have already mentioned the Paris psychosomatic school and especially the autism research following Tustin.

Freud had observed that if memories become conscious once more, they exhibit no sensory quality (see above; 1900a, 540). However, the sensualisation of such presentations is normally possible for the personality. But what if this regredient process is disturbed? Bion had observed that there are elements that are not transformed into α-elements, remain raw or as β-elements. They are not capable of stable connection, can temporarily stick together, sometimes clump together with the inclusion of α-elements to form bizarre objects. These elements have no psychic quality, but do they have sensual quality? How then is the relationship between sensual and psychic quality to be determined? Is it not absurd to claim that elements that originally have raw sensuality are not sensual when the transformation fails?

If we go into the traumatic realm in the narrower sense (in which non-existence and breakdown are included), the answer is clear – they must not have any sensual quality, otherwise there is an immediate threat of retraumatisation, even more: The core realm in the narrower sense is without any sensual quality, not even ordered according to pleasure-unpleasure. In contrast, autistic/autistoid as well as psychosomatic disorders, which belong more to the envelopment, are by definition sensual-bodily: Autistic objects and forms are self-created sensual states; psychosomatic symptoms express themselves on the body. But, paradoxically, these are almost always without a sensually differentiated quality.

Two short examples: When I was sent as a student to a boy with severe autistic disorders, he did not respond to any offer from me, not even the greeting was returned. He completely dismantled cassette recorders, then screwed them back together in a flash, hour after hour, day after day. Desperate and totally helpless, I did the same – dilettantishly, I admit. So we sat next to each other. I immersed myself

DOI: 10.4324/9781003434207-5

in his world, enveloped in mechanical activity, the world as if behind a curtain, very far away.[1] I felt the second skin, the distance of the world, the material, the shapes everything, but everything without a conscious sensual quality!

Many pain patients are almost never able to describe their pain. They say: "The shoulder hurts" or "It hurts there." When they do describe sensual impressions, they are usually assumed "qualities": "Yes, yes, it's a pulling pain." If one then asks whether it is a pressing or stabbing pain, they again answer affirmatively. Kütemeyer (e.g. 2003), a psychosomatic therapist from Cologne, in cooperation with linguists, has developed a technique that opens up a narrative space so that patients dare to describe their pain. Staying close to the sensual, using images, paying attention to sound and rhythm, the therapists meet the patients. The patients feel that the subject is really listening and begin to tell. For example, a patient with severe shoulder pain was able to describe her pain in this encouraged way: "It stings like it did when my mother stuck the knife in my shoulder...."

These, for example, enveloping, billowing, armoured, solidified, hardened states are thus without differentiated sensual quality. How can this be? The thesis was that raw sensual elements accumulate in the pre-conception and become psychic with realisation. If this process fails, β-elements remain. Why do β-elements not have a differentiated sensual quality? I suspect for two reasons: First, differentiated sensual quality in the mental system could be linked to psychic qualities, e.g. sensual characteristics such as tender, warm, melting with the psychic quality "to love". On the other hand, β-elements are not connectable, which makes differentiation enormously difficult. Then sensual qualities exist only rudimentarily.

This derivation from a clinical observation could confirm Bion's thesis, which he made for hallucinosis, namely, that the mental event which is transformed into a sense impression provides pleasure or pain (Bion, 1970, 37), but does not lead into sensual differentiation.

This makes the advice on technique from autism research more comprehensible: e.g. to make the patient's descriptions more precise by reformulating and paraphrasing; to give expression to experience[2]; to give "hey" interpretations (Alvarez, 2012) that vitalise and allow another to emerge; to formulate closely oriented to experience; to use imitative co-movements to grasp the inner worlds[3]; to circumscribe perceived states and excitations; to offer hunches as transitory statements (Bion, 1975); to bring together scattered sensations; to avoid overwhelming self-object determinations (e.g. use of the third person) and symbolic levels, etc.

We can thus not only confirm our statement made above that in the nameless the elements are not only not psychically qualified, but confirm that they are also sensually stripped (s. ch. 2.5), but also derive treatment-related consequences: The sensualisation of the nameless core complex is not possible for the patients; the core of the nameless is not sensual. The perverse-autistoid defence only proceeds according to pleasure or pain, is without differentiated sensual qualities. But the regredient sensualisation of elements is important for the analytic cure, also because it serves the objectal hope. Even more, without the sensual level, a grasp of psychic reality is not possible.

Does this position not collide with Bion's renunciation of memory, desire and understanding?

4.2 Encountering the nameless in holding

In a repressed dynamic, the defended complex can be clearly felt as resistance from a certain point onwards (this is why Freud attached such great importance to resistance, especially transference-resistance). The defences are also more or less clearly discernible. I.e. the defences are related as psychic formations to the repressed conflict, which can be sensed as a contoured complex.

In the case of a nameless dynamic, the situation is quite different: The actual complex, the encapsulation, only exists like a kind of background noise, a contoured idea of the content does not – and cannot – exist. Entropic fragments, nothingness, emptiness, even the traumatic actual has no contour, not even a sensual contour.

But that's not all: The classical defences (repression; rationalisation; projection; introjection; inversion into the opposite, etc.) refer to the defenced – and in relation to the object ("I resist you, object! I won't show it to you"). The perverse excitations and the autistoid rumination and freezing as defensive formations do not refer or cannot be decoded to the encapsulated contents – and have no relationship to the object!

The complete lack of contours of the core complex and the fact that the defence formations do not refer to it, in the absence of the objectal reference and the deficient sensualisation of elements and states, now pose challenges to the method and the methodology of psychoanalysis in nameless states. Free-floating attention and free association function, among other things, through the progressive emergence of presentations (descendants) and the regredient sensualisation of these presentations. Both are not present in the nameless in the classical sense. How should this impossibility be dealt with?

Bion's no memory, no desire, no understanding, which for me represent an important deepening of free-floating attention, aim, among other things, at not being blinded by a sensually saturated knowledge.

> Memory and desire exercise and intensify those aspects of the mind that derive from sensuous experience. They thus promote capacity derived from sense impressions and designed to serve impressions of sense. They deal respectively with sense impressions of what is supposed to have happened and sense impressions of what has not yet happened.
>
> (Bion, 1967a, 136)

We can add understanding here: Memory refers primarily to the past, desire to the future and understanding to a present understanding that believes it can recognise psychic reality from sensual experiences. In psychoanalysis, this form of using memory, desire and understanding is a defence against grasping psychic reality, a countertransference in the narrower sense. For Bion, they correspond to posses-siveness and sensuous greed (Bion, 1970, 33). I think there are also other mecha-nisms at play, such as anal domination and control.

But without sensual impressions and sensations, psychoanalytic work is not pos-sible and understanding is impossible. This is how I also understand Bion, who "obscurely" (Winnicott) states:

> Memory and desire are essential elements in the composition of the new for-mulation, but a distinction must be made between two classes of mental event. One is an evocation of memory and desire with impulses of possessiveness and sensuous greed: the impulses generate memory and desire; memory and desire generate sensuous greed. The other is the evocation of memories and desires because the experience of at-one-ment resembles possession and sensuous ful-filment. The classes differ because the mode of selection differs, and since the classes differ the interpretation (the formulation by the analyst) will differ. The evocation of that which provided a container for possessions, and of the sensu-ous gratifications with which to fill it, will differ from an evocation stimulated by at-one-ment. The exercises in discarding memory and desire must be seen as preparatory to a state of mind in which O can evolve. The facilitation of "constellation" must in turn be seen as a step in the process of at-one-ment (the transformation O → K). In practice this means not that the analyst recalls some relevant memory but that a relevant constellation will be evoked during the process of at-one-ment with O, the process denoted by transformation O → K.
>
> (Bion, 1970, 33)

Now we have a remarkable situation before us: nameless states that are signif-icantly lacking in sensuality, with a vital need for sensual orientation.[4] Without sensual attachment, we cannot orient ourselves in the world. This also applies to psychoanalysts.

Patients need help to grasp their experience in a sensually differentiated way. In my opinion, it is important that this process is oriented towards the patient's experience.

That is, the patient must be able to arrive at his sensual qualifications, which are not determined by saturated knowledge of the object. There is a great danger, for example, of qualifying a coprophilia too quickly as smelly, greasy, repulsive, etc., and thus overlooking the second-skin character. The sensual qualification should start from the basal distinction Lust-Unlust, pleasure and pain. The objectal dimen-sion is important here: If we refrain from too early, saturated determination of the sensual, contrary to expectation the patient feels held, seen and can build up his own sensual differentiations.

But gentleness is also of great importance for the analyst: We have to find a way to the psychic reality of the patient in the relationship, which we cannot and may not determine. Correctly sensually defined and alphabetised elements help in grasping this psychic reality. (If we overlook, for example, the two-skin character of coprophilia, we may miss the patient.)

With this we may have found a first idea for approaching nameless states: Start from the most rudimentary sensuality and from there begin a sensualisation. The careful determination and differentiation that the analytic pair undertakes release dreaming processes and give space for the (re)establishment of objectal hope. If we return to our basic theoretical model, the dynamic-structural process becomes more understandable. The pre-conception that must be reactivated is that of the breast. The sensual elements must accumulate in it. Just as the sensual hunger of the infant accumulates in the pre-conception, the sensual elements created by the couple now connect with the pre-conception. The differentiated sensual elements have emerged in the transference process, and are suitable for the pre-conception.

If we take these considerations as a basis, holding is of great importance in this phase. Briefly, my conceptualisation of holding (which differs from Winnicott's).[5]

In the first phase of its life, the child is maximally dependent; Winnicott calls it absolute dependence.

> In this state the infant has no means of knowing about the maternal care, which is largely a matter of prophylaxis. He cannot gain control over what is well and what is badly done, but is only in a position to gain profit or to suffer disturbance.
> (Winnicott, 1960, 590)

Holding for Winnicott is psychological and physiological holding; both forms are indistinguishable for the child. However, Winnicott gives preference to physical holding: "Holding includes especially the physical holding of the infant, which is a form of loving. It is perhaps the only way in which a mother can show the infant her love of it" (Winnicott, 1960, 592) – a view that I cannot share and which, in my opinion, is not empirically tenable. Severe disturbances in holding lead to states of annihilation that interrupt the going on being: "Being and annihilation are the two alternatives. The holding environment therefore has as its main function the reduction to a minimum of impingements to which the infant must react with resultant annihilation of personal being" (Winnicott, 1960, 591; also in 1965; see also various other works in 1965). From absolute dependence develops relative dependence. "Here the infant can become aware of the need for the details of maternal care, and can to a growing extent relate them to personal impulse, and then later, in a psycho-analytic treatment, can reproduce them in the transference" (Winnicott 1960, 591). The mother later emerges as a real object for the infant. Winnicott locates disturbances in these processes with the object, but they act as threats to personal self-existence of the infant.

Holding is inextricably linked to "primary maternal preoccupation":

> The mother who develops this state that I have called "primary maternal preoccupation" provides a setting for the infant's constitution to begin to make itself evident, for the developmental tendencies to start to unfold, and for the infant to experience spontaneous movement and *become the owner of the sensations* that are appropriate to this early phase of life.
> (Winnicott, 1975 [1956], 303; italics BN)

Winnicott now assumes that this early situation can be restored in the analytic treatment. The analyst, however, can now act as a caring, empathic and resonant object with the patient's needs, thus enabling a repair, subsequent integration and psychic growth.

If we equate holding environment with the analytic attitude of meeting the patient psychically and sensually in reverie (primary maternal preoccupation) and, together with him, to sensualise undifferentiated impressions and sensations again in a differentiated way, thus reactivating psychic functions and establishing relationship, then we come closer to an important attitude which, in my opinion, is indicated for patients with nameless states.

In my understanding, holding is a recurring posture (also in the analytic process), at the same time a necessary first reaction to fears of disintegration. Instinctively we take our child, who is in fear of disintegration, in our arms, find the right posture, the right "pressure," the right pitch of voice, etc. – and hold until we feel almost by the change in our child's muscular tension that it feels held, is with itself again and finally can perceive the object/the world again. Annihilation is double to think of – the feeling of falling apart physically and falling psychically. Holding the first emergency therapy.

In psychoanalysis, such holding is not a concrete physical one, but shows up in the attitude of the analyst who can "stay integrated," who can hold dissolving states in himself and in the transference. In my experience, patients with nameless states test over many months whether they can hope that the analyst can hold the nameless when it occurs.[6]

This form of holding shows itself above all in the attitude of the analyst, wanting to be there, and the readiness becomes perceptible to face the unknown, which, as already written, is present as a kind of background radiation. This total situation can certainly be interpreted, interpretations in which we address, as it were, the "non-existent," the "negative."

Although the nameless is inconceivable, "something" in the patients is permanently occupied with it. This shows itself atmospherically in the treatment. In contact, the patients seem, for example, like someone we are talking to, but who is waiting the whole time for an important phone call, or is constantly looking at the clock because he has to leave. An irritation that can be addressed in a noticing (not evaluating!) way ("Somehow it sometimes seems as if one part is not really here, busy with something else") and is heard objectally by patients. Also by addressing the atmospherically dark, empty, nothingness, we bring ourselves into play as a holding object ("It seems as if there is something very dark in the background"). Another technical method is to experience that the interpsychic communication fails. After all, patients feel that what they want to communicate does not connect psychically. For example, in the case of a hypochondriac patient who speaks of fear of death without succeeding in touching the object, the following intervention may be indicated:

There is a threat, but it is probably not in the body, but in your soul. But one more thing strikes me: You cannot feel or sense this threat. But I know how awful it must be to try to communicate such a threat, then feel the other person doesn't understand it.

We acknowledge the threat and locate it. And we find the courage to say (which is always agonisingly grasped by those affected anyway) that we cannot feel their communications, but communicate that we know the horror of such enclosure.

In my opinion, such interventions are holding interpretations. They address the "absence," the void, on several levels: an unnamable core threat; being occupied by the nameless; the experience that the desperate attempts to communicate the threat fail; the experience of being lonely and cut off from the objects. Holding expresses itself in wanting to see the distress, the threat, and to be there. In such holding, we emerge as an object that can notice the sensual, imaginative and objectal absence – thus creating a first objectal bridge.

In my experience, holding dominates the first phase of work with people who have nameless states within them. The sensual differentiation of sensations and impressions, the holding interpretations have the one aim of generating elements that release further material and dynamise the process. But the other effect (especially on the part of the patients) is the development and testing of the object relationship, whether it can exist in holding and finally become containing. Then the nameless can show itself in a moment of presence. In my opinion, it is important to keep the free-floating attention, herein no memory, no desire and no understanding. Winnicott, here rather following Ferenczi, argues against the analytic ideal of abstinence. I believe that this is not only incorrect, but dangerous. Either it creates artefacts, especially transference cures (in the negative sense), or it leads to uncertainties in the boundaries that are fundamentally important for patients.

Even though it may seem that the holding phase in analytic work is relatively clear, this impression is deceptive. It is not only about nameless dynamics, but about the whole spectrum of analytic work: Besides nameless states and their complex defensive fortresses, conflicts play a role, symbolic levels, paranoid-schizoid and depressive dynamics, acting out, enactment, resistances, transference-resistances, etc., etc. These different dynamics are also not neatly sorted as in a layer model, but are pushed into each other, partly only recognisable afterwards (nachträglich).[7] Working on these repressed (in the broad sense) contents is also important for nameless dynamics: It promotes the trust that an object wants to understand and neither just jumps at the "nameless" nor avoids it, i.e. gives in to its fear of "what is to come."

I see one of the greatest challenges for the treatment of nameless states in this complexity, in which a wide variety of dynamics are at work at once in almost every sequence of treatment and which cannot be determined in the here and now but can often only be roughly ordered afterwards.

I would first like to demonstrate this problem with a detailed example.[8]

V On the treatment technique for nameless dynamics – a detailed case study

A patient comes forward saying he suffers from "severe skin cancer fears, everything examined, always without findings." He has a real fear of death. Rationally, he knows this is "hypochondriac nonsense, but the certainty that I will die remains." He has had these fears "for many months" after seeing "a picture of the battered torso of a 'dead torture victim.'"

The statement is, typical of hypochondria, quite confusing: mortal fear of an incurable cancer for which there are no medical findings, but the certified absence of findings does not reassure, the fear remains. Untypical, on the other hand, was the indicative statement ("certainty, I'm going to die"), which in itself would scare "hypochondriacs" too much. The trigger, the image of the torture victim, also did not strike me as typically hypochondriacal.

He was the child of a young, drug-addicted mother who came from a well-off family. His father was unknown. Since his birth, he had repeatedly come to his grandparents, and his mother had tried to withdraw from drugs. He then returned, mostly to desolate conditions. Shortly before he was five years old, he was "taken away" from his mother and came to live permanently with his grandparents. The mother later died under unexplained circumstances. He himself never found contact with his peers, was an outsider, bullied, spat on, beaten. His scientific talent "saved" him.

The suspicion was that these might be nameless states: Early, presumably cumulative traumatisation, hypochondriacal autistoid symptoms, atmospheric impressions gave rise to this suspicion.

The treatment[9] began taciturnly and never became wordy. After about three or four months, the patient remarked: "My girlfriend broke up with me because of my depression. Seven months again. Seems 'a magic number.'"

I noticed in two places. A worry sounded in a distant echo: The magical seven months are halfway around in treatment. Will the analyst also give up with the taciturn patient whom it is difficult to understand? Should this barely perceptible transference have been interpreted? If so, how? Focusing on the object ("You wonder if I too could give up after seven months...")? Or focusing on fear ("You are afraid that the relationship won't last here either...")? But does this objectal perspective capture the patient, what is happening? If we use Ferro's "trick," no dream emerges: "I dreamt: My girlfriend broke up with me because of my depression. Seven months again. Seems a magic number."

The statement does not visualise...

To me, this concern also seemed too quiet in the session; I listened at the phrase "because of my depression." I felt the patient did not understand these words.

I would encourage him to narrate and asked what exactly had happened. He elaborated that his girlfriend said that she had not found him, that she was so sorry.

While this statement touches me, the patient seems as if he does not know what his girlfriend is talking about. But what does that mean? Has the patient heard the affective, sad-painful content of his girlfriend's statement, communicated it to me, but immediately rejected it in a splitting manner? Or has the patient not heard this emotional dimension, is it my addition, my empathic interpretation? In any case, an emotional-sensual dimension emerges via the girlfriend that seems closer, more accessible to me; for I say benevolently-spontaneously: "That sounds different from 'because of my depression'. She was looking for you, not finding you."

"That's right," he confirms thoughtfully. I mean to sense how something about my words seems to engage him.

How does he hear the intervention? In solidarity with the girlfriend, perhaps even reproachfully persecuting: His girlfriend is looking for him, his analyst is looking for him; both of them can't find him, give him up? Or does he even sense the opposite position: His analyst is looking for him and discovers a connection between depression and suffering/searching and not finding, which the patient does not feel – which would be a first finding? In the first case it would be more of a paranoid-schizoid dynamic, in the second case an emergence in which an object seeks him and connections between depression and suffering, seeking/not-finding. But it is also possible that none of these perspectives is already valid, the patient is in a completely self-referential state.

First of all, it seems important to me that the patient seems thoughtful. It fits with this that after a pause he says: "But you also use the word 'loneliness'!" This sentence does not sound like a reply, but like a "nonunderstanding question mark." I therefore tell him that then the word loneliness does not meet his sensibilities any more than depression seems to him to be connectable with suffering, searching and not finding.
"I don't know what loneliness is…," he resigns.

In my opinion, not only are many perspectives on the material conceivable, but they could run parallel: The continuing concern that time will pass in the analysis, that the analyst will give up; the awareness that words like loneliness and depression do not capture his experience; the pressure to conform to the analyst's language game; a certain irritation at not understanding, at not getting it right; an acting out to avoid the experience of separation, of being separate, which then leads circularly to the patient feeling increasingly abandoned in the session, etc.

But I perceived another dynamic more clearly in the material, namely, a person for whom the psychic and a receptive object are alien in wide areas, who tries within himself to grasp these dimensions, experiences painfully that he reaches his limits here. But although he can hardly think, the object, emotional and sensual dimensions have become accessible.

I therefore say that words like loneliness, depression are quite foreign to him, but that he is perceptibly preoccupied by the fact that someone has sought him and not found him. "Exactly," he confirms.

This interpretation takes up some of the technical recommendations that have been developed in recent years, such as formulating in an experience-oriented way, paraphrasing perceived excitations, refraining from overburdening self-object determinations (hence the use of the third person) and avoiding symbolic levels. The most important aspect of such interpretations, however, is that we emerge as an object who seeks to understand the patient's inner world, who communicates what he perceives, e.g. that complex concepts are foreign to him, and who senses that something has occupied and touched him. Indirectly, the dimensions that move more in the psychic-objectal space are also addressed in this way. In this way, hopes for objectal structures can slowly emerge.

Months later, I experienced the relationship as more sustained, he confided in me how he had sometimes been brutally beaten up by classmates, why was never clear to him, and how once, as if that was not enough, a teacher humiliated him. This teacher forced him to go to his tormentor, who had maltreated him with kicks when he was already lying on the ground, and to "get along," thereby making the patient the culprit. "My body was covered with bruises and I was forced by the teacher and in his presence to hold out my hand, which he refused to do." He was able to describe these scenes densely and realistically with his capacity for hyperrealistic perception, so that *for me* his experience was very accessible. He could also, *it seemed to me*, react very adequately and sensitively to my words.

He was silent for a very long time, I asked him where he was.

Reluctantly, he replied, "At the light play." (Light play is his term for tree-shadow structures projected by the sun on the wall above the couch.)

I said he seemed like he was completely immersed in that world. "No, I'm not. Not now that you're talking," he said sternly.

I abruptly felt harshly rejected and asked if I had pulled him out of the immersion.

"I am not immersed, I am one with it, no: I am. Don't you understand that? You don't get it!"

"Then help me."

Silence. "Just leave it!"

"It's hard for me to understand. You were able to communicate yourself and your terrible experiences so densely and understandably, there was something shared..."

"There was nothing shared, you just don't get it."

In the next session he hastened to emphasise, sincerely and seriously, that for him there had been nothing common, shared. I felt that this was true, but I did not understand. I also told him that. Over the next few weeks, we tried again and again to understand this situation. In this context, it came to light how much violence there had been. His mother kept bringing junkies into the small flat; there was frequent sexual and physical violence. Drugs, violence, unresponsive mother, he cried out from hunger, from fear, from neglect until the neighbours called the police, who sometimes found him alone. Then he would once again come to the grandparents.

Thus we could reconstruct with some evidence (see Freud, 1937d) that the confusing treatment situation was perhaps a repetition of early experiences. As a small child, he sought the closeness of his beaten, battered mother, still dazed by drugs and alcohol, believing that he was tenderly there for her. Perhaps the mother even spoke to herself as if in shock, but did not notice him at all or only as a self-object. When she then registered him, he was harshly, brutally rejected by her. In other words, an early scene that accelerated the abandonment of hope for a holding, loving object, which was finally cumulatively absorbed into the nameless. This objectal abandonment was restaged in the treatment in a role reversal.

But how could this scene be conceptualised?

One possibility, which I also thought I sensed, could be the following: The patient came into an actual condition via the narration of the school violence, i.e. the experiences were felt as actual, hardly located in the past. In this actual condition, an adhesive two-dimensionality spread. That is, in the role reversal, there was no identification with the mother, but an adhesive equation of the maltreated mother and the beaten schoolboy. In the narration of the humiliating school violence, he became the mother adhesively, no longer perceiving the empathetic analyst. This adhesive equation led to the patient's experience that there was no common ground, nothing shared between us. In this condition he became entangled in the light play, i.e. it became an autistoid form (autistic form, see Tustin, 1984). Then my asking ("Where are you?") would be a destruction of the autistoid form, the patient reacts with corresponding aversion. Here his harsh form is not a rejection of an object, but arousal rage/anxiety, because the autistoid form in his experience has been destroyed.

But another possibility cannot be ruled out: For the patient, the school violence is no longer a remembered story, but an actual event. He gets into an adhesive two-dimensional state, glues himself to the play of light. With my address, an object reappears for him in which he quickly places projectively dependent, needy, hurt, searching parts, which he then brutally rejects. Since I was in the position of the little child, I thought I was close to him and had to experience the rejection first hand. In this perspective, an autistoid dynamic would have turned into an objectal one in a flash.

We can see here how difficult it is clinically-empirically to differentiate autistoid and objectal dynamics, adhesive equations, identifications, entanglements, transference enactments. The aporia, that is, the determination of whether the dynamic is an autistoid one or one that fluctuates between autistoid and paranoid-schizoid, is not decidable in the treatment situation, but also not really resolvable afterwards (nachträglich). Why did I not interpret the destructive? Or why did I not technically intervene in a trauma-therapeutic way (e.g. calling for pauses)? I don't know, but I suspect that I preconsciously perceived the actual in the material.

The autistoid may dominate in the treatment, but objectal dynamics exist interwoven and then lead in the further course into a common search process, even if this remains – quasi as a protection against too much relationship – in the reconstructive.

Perhaps it was such reconstructions that finally made it possible for him to tell something he had never said before. When he was four, almost five years old, after a loud tumult in the flat and after it had become "completely quiet," he ventured out of his room to look for his mother. He found her naked, beaten almost to death by one of her many "lovers," "lifeless in blood and vomit." Haematomas, bruises, injuries, vomit everywhere. He ran back, crawled into bed, cowered under the covers "for hours."

He came to live with his grandparents. To this day he doesn't know where his mother had gone, no one talked about it. He never saw her again. He never dared to ask because he felt "guilty about my mother's death." In my opinion, this is *not* a memory, but a traumatic actual event that the patient has kept within himself all his life. For whatever reason, the image of the torture victim released processes of disengagement that he had to master. The adhesive equation: battered mother – torture victim – skin cancer was a defence against the breakdown in which hypochondria was not primarily a substitute capsule for released nameless contents (its primary function in hypochondriacal dynamics), but a second skin, even if it was a tribute to the Super-Ego (Bion).

A moment of presence creates a shared understanding and a deep libidinal relationship between the participants, which are important for the following dynamics. This was also the case here; the patient felt understood. Although the presence moment created relationship, lifted much into the namable, tangibly important things about the nameless remained uncomprehended. It even seemed to spread. A paralysing melancholy gripped everything, which I could not put into words. I could not find a way to the patient. Yet he expressed his experience depressingly: "The darkness spreads more and more, soon everything will be extinguished."

When I opened the window of the practice before a session with the patient in this condition, I saw the whole cornucopia of the splendour of spring. Then Heiner Müller's remark about the shameless green of the trees popped into my head. Heiner Müller could still perceive the shameless green of the trees after his devastating diagnosis, i.e. he was still connected to the world in fear, despair and envy – not even this rest remained for the patient. There was nothing left with him, no more connection to the world, to the objects.

I was able to tell the patient that. He remained silent, then suddenly sat up, fearing he would get a panic attack.

The traumatic image of the mother "beaten to death" can be sublated in the moment of presence. It contains a traumatic rigidity that the patient calls "guilt," which can only be bound adhesively-hypochondrically. One can now understand the following dynamic in treatment as a melancholic one, as Freud (1917e) described it, in which the "shadow of the object" falls on the patient and leads into darkness. This dynamic, which I understand as autistoid in its most severe forms (see Nissen, 2016), plays a role without question. But the experienced scene has also connected with his dying off in the earliest days of childhood, so it is a first retrospective (nachträgliche) form in which the breakdown emerges that occurred for the patient but was not experienced. For in first moment of presence, the namelessness of one's own dying was not sublated. This darkness was not only there, but spread out threateningly, leading everything into extinction. It was possible to discover this with Heiner Müller's line and to offer it to the patient. *Only in the relationship could it become real and be sublated in the presentative.* That is, my becoming aware of the extinction of all psychic with the help of Heiner Müller's art enabled the *emergence of a pre-conception*, which was then *realised in the relationship* and *psychically qualified the experience*. The moment of presence thus does not emerge in my evidence, but only in the relationship. This becoming real is a joint discovery, a creation and subjugation of the couple. At the same time, the analyst becomes the witness and preserver of this becoming-real: There is an object that knows about this being dead and has sublated and preserved it within itself – an important factor in such treatments.

4.3 Noticing, transformation and caesura in nameless dynamics

In my opinion, very different clinical dynamics can be observed in the case study, which I would like to discuss briefly.

In the classical attitude of free-floating attention, I hear the patient's statement that after seven months the girlfriend has broken up. De facto, my noticing guides me through the scene. My listening to the phrase "because of my depression" leads to the encouragement of a narrative deepening, which the patient also does. With my spontaneity and with my words that trigger emotions ("wanted," "not found") I reformulate. The patient reacts thoughtfully, which I notice in the steady hovering. He expresses his non-understanding of separation and "depression" through the communication that the analyst is talking about loneliness. In a normal conversation, his idea would probably have been disturbing, but in the basic analytical stance, an intuitive connection succeeds: He seems to have made an effort to find words (depression) that he believes the analyst understands. However, he himself does not seem to have any words to express the experience of his world. With his formulation ("But you also use the word 'loneliness'") he reveals himself and indirectly invokes the object, even trusts that the object can digest the irritating leap in conversation. I add a transitory interpretation, point out that the words loneliness and depression do not represent his sensations, that his world of experience is not represented in my language game ("Sprachspiel"). He confirms.

The scene seems harmless, but in my opinion it is not. It points to a caesura. Bion writes, choosing an extreme example to illustrate his thoughts, that the "analyst cannot interpret the 'sights' a foetus could 'see' if subjected to pressure on the optic pits" (1975, 40). From which world does my patient speak? Only from one in which he lacks definitional hypotheses? Or from one in which he not only cannot understand anything, but is also not allowed to understand anything, even though he has "sights"? It seems important to me that the caesura is not overcome – and cannot be overcome. But it emerges in the relationship.

How profound, how fundamental this caesura is then becomes subsequently perceptible in the scene in which the patient describes the humiliating school violence. It is "only" his autistoid-perverse defence that flares up, but the actuality, the two-dimensionality and the second-skin formation become accessible. My mistake was probably that I understood his descriptions as past events, assumed that this past had gone through transformations and was represented. That is why I thought we were in contact. But for the patient, the past was present, so much so that he had to spin himself into an autistoid form. He expressed how he experiences (non-)relationship – in the adhesive equation as disturbing, in the objectal hope as devastating rejection. I.e. with my desire and memory assumptions I fell out of free-floating attention without realising it.

But could I have interpreted what the patient was experiencing if I had been able to maintain my attitude? I believe such scenes are aporetic in nature.

Schneider has addressed the issue of aporia in several works (2006, 2007, 2014), separating it from Socratic (see 2007, 658f). He defines aporia "from the Greek aporí a: hopelessness, impassability, distress, doubt" (2007, 657) and has examined it for objectal dynamics on several levels, e.g. related to transference and resistance, countertransference and acting out, but also to the negative therapeutic response, the danger of healing, as well as to the frame, the interpretation, the third position and the analytic couple. He writes:

"Analysing as an analytic practice is essentially aporetic in nature and consists to a significant extent in resolving and transforming aporetic constellations in an analytic way…" (2006, 900).

Analysing as an analytic practice is essentially aporetic. The resolution of an aporetic situation cannot be achieved in a methodical, purposeful way … it is rather a creative act of the analytic couple. … [It] *consists in this respect in the attempt to emerge analytically from the aporetic trench, to transform the aporetic constellation.*

(2006, 903)

"Lapidary paradox" puts it: "*Analysing consists in making analysing possible*" (2006, 903). He also derives from this the necessity of an "error culture" (2014).
Reik wrote as early as 1932 (!):

It has to be said more than once – you have to say it three times – that the non-understanding of a psychological connection means progress compared to a superficial understanding. While that understanding is like landing in a dead end, this non-understanding leaves all kinds of possibilities open.

(Reik 1932, 15; translation BN)

And Bion writes: "In analysis it is recovery from the unfortunate decision, the use of the mistaken decision that we have to accustom ourselves to deal with" (1975, 44).
My hopelessness in the scene was total. I had not grasped the scene, not understood it. I had sensed that the play of light had become an autistoid form, but did not even come to the intuitive bifurcation of whether it could have been an autistoid or a violent projective-objectal dynamic. I merely tried to bring myself in as an object that, even though my psychoanalytic thinking was knocked out, continued to try to understand what did not seem understandable.
In this case, the non-understanding, which I do not want to relativise or even elevate to a technique (!), led to a productive process in which, in a moment of presence, the connection between the mother who was beaten almost to death, the torture victim and the skin cancer could become. Here, via a transformation into a presence moment (O), something of the dead happens that the patient, when he found his mother, had already suffered! The breakdown from the earliest days has revealed itself here retrospectively (nachträglich), a situation that finally arrested being dead as a child. However, being dead has not yet shown itself in this moment of presence, but rather its helpless attempts to survive in lulling hypochondria. But with it, being dead found its announcement.
In consequence, everything threatened to go out. The tremendously precise sentence that takes one's breath away: "The darkness spreads more and more, soon everything is extinguished" was not in the objectal, but could still connect with Heiner Müller's line. It was possible to bring this feeling of being gripped into the

treatment. This is how the moment of presence came about, in which being dead, the loss of everything, could be there, and life dawned in the opposite direction.

This moment of presence *is* a caesura, not unlike the example chosen by Bion (with reference to Freud) of pre- and postnatal, namely, being dead – life.

Since my reading of Bion's "caesura" differs from the widely accepted readings today, I will briefly explain my understanding.

To be clear, I assume that Bion introduces the term "caesura" to describe O and in particular the transformation into O from another vertex. He is trying to describe the analytical attitude that is necessary to make O possible and (hopefully) to understand it, but in particular to grasp, or give us an inkling of, the unknown of both the states to be transformed and the states that are transformed.

In my opinion, Bion wants to point out that there are states and processes that differ so much from a "normal" understanding that they appear as if they do not exist. He chooses the image of birth (prenatal – postnatal). There are things that suggest feelings that could be described as love, hate, etc., but which seem to have such an intense and unformed character (38) that these processes would perhaps be better described in anatomical, somatic or physiological terms. I.e. there could be processes from a world, "which are in the womb of time eventually show themselves in the conscious life of the person concerned who then has to act in the situation which has now become actual" (Bion, 1975, 43) It is difficult to grasp this, even in psychoanalytic encounters:

> … but what may appeal to the human mind because it seems to be logical, or to fit in with such powers of logic as we have, may be by no means the correct interpretation of the factual situation which is beyond our comprehension or experience. To distort that experience in order to make it fit into such capacities as we have is a dangerous thing….. The analyst has to use what we hope is a non-pathological method of splitting because the total situation that presents itself to us is beyond our capacity, just as we suppose that it is beyond the capacity of the infant to have a grasp of the world as we know it as adults. It is natural for the infant to see a *part* of the world of reality; that particular view is not wrong – it is inadequate. To limit ourselves to the observation only of what we understand is denying ourselves the raw material on which present and possibly future wisdom and knowledge might depend. The fact that it is incomprehensible now, because our minds are unsuitable or ill-fitted to grasp it, is not a reason for limiting the facts such as are actually available.
>
> (Bion, 1975, 45–46)

I.e. we have to attune ourselves[10] in our attitude to states, procedures and processes that lie beyond what can be expected, beyond our previous understanding. This applies above all to nameless states that lie beyond the psychic. We do not know them, cannot know them and will not know them in the future – they lie beyond our experiences and expectations.

Bion still gives advice for interpreting: The interpretation has to be made at the right moment; it is, therefore, necessary that this non-pathological splitting, ordering of those splits and choice of formulation become part of a rapid and practised mind (Bion, 1975, 41).[11] It is astonishing to me that Bion does not refer at this point to the transformation in O, which in my opinion is the only event in the analytic relationship in which the caesura becomes investigable in statu nascendi. Instead, Bion gives advice in the quotation that is not appropriate to the complexity of the situation; indeed, it seems impractical to me. The interpretation of the moment of presence and the transformation into the presentative are primordial processes, with the characteristics of discovery, creation and subjugation.

Bion now points to an aspect that seems important to me in presence moments that acquire the characteristics of a caesura, even if it is difficult to understand. It concerns a form of bidirectionality:

> In the psychoanalytic experience we are concerned both with the translation in the direction of what we do not know into something which we do know or which we can communicate, and also from what we do know and can communicate to what we do not know and are not aware of because it is unconscious...
>
> (Bion, 1975, 47)

Bion relates this consideration to psyche – soma – states. Rational-causal thinking people, since they are at home in the world of things, could express psychic processes as physical in their rational form of communication and thus bring psychic into their because-logic, since they only experience physical.

I am now interested in this bidirectionality above all for the moment of presence and the transformation into the presentative.

The nameless is not psychic, not conscious and not unconscious. It happens in the relationship in the moment of presence, is to be grasped in the Pcpt/Cs. It is a circular paradoxical state. The unknown, that is, what the analysand and the analysed do not know, is sublated into a presentative symbol, which means translated into something we know. We now know it in three forms: The nameless is sublated in the presentative symbol – in the sublated it has become conception, transformed overcome, but also remained nameless.

At the same time, however, what the analyst and the analysand know becomes something they do not know at the moment of presence. That means two things: The knowledge (K) that has accumulated in the run-up is deleted in the moment of presence, is no longer known. And the nameless that happens in the moment and what the couple knew becomes unconscious, must become part of emerging thing presentations, connectable with the word presentations emerging in the presentative.

It has to become conscious as well as unconscious so that both systems, Ucs as well as Pcs/Cs, can work binocularly on the processing, the digestion of the nameless – and find forms to pacify the non-transformable part in such a way that it loses its horror – mostly at least.

Bion translates Freud's famous sentence: "There is much more continuity between intra-uterine life and earliest infancy than the impressive caesura[1] of the act of birth would have us believe." As per Freud (1926d, 138): "There is much more continuity between autonomically appropriate quanta and the waves of conscious thought and feeling than the impressive caesura of transference and countertransference would have us believe" (49). Freud, however, continues:

> What happens is that the child's biological situation as a foetus is replaced for it by a psychical object-relation to its mother. But we must not forget that during its intra-uterine life the mother was not an object for the foetus, and that at that time there were no objects at all.
>
> (1926d, 138)

We must also think of the nameless and the name found as a continuum, but we may hope that the caesura of the moment of presence that takes place in the relationship enables psychic growth.

4.4   On living in the nameless

Strictly speaking, every moment of presence represents a caesura, since the transformation (better: sublation) that has occurred creates a before and after. But some moments of presence really do acquire an existential dimension, not inferior to the examples chosen by Bion (1975): from non-existence to existence, from no-being to being, from two-dimensionality into relational space. The fundamental difference between the being-on-the-world/being-in-the-world of people who have psychic representations and those who live in nameless states becomes conceivable.

How does it feel to live in a world in which the nameless is like a black hole, in which a breakdown has taken place?[12] One can understand a breakdown, an early traumatic event that interrupts the going on being, as a malignant caesura. How does a small child experience it? How does an adult experience it? Like someone who has found the courage to enter into an analytic relationship? How does the experience change when the nameless has been sublated in a moment of presence? As analysts, we can gain some knowledge from the moment a patient enters treatment.

Let's look at the two detailed examples from this point of view. I don't know, I think, to this day how, for example, my patient experienced her life before she slipped into coprophilic stupor. Atmospherically, I could sense something of her experience after she had met the sex-addicted man: She encountered the incarnation of the death drive, probably suspected that she was getting too close to the black hole, saved herself into a senseless world of autistoid-perverse acting. This world blew at me in dark forebodings, e.g. in the nothingness that arose when she spoke of the nocturnal car journeys. The sensuality, the sensualisation of the non-sensual coprophilia became a milestone: The patient transferred the presentation of having had her excrement in her hands to the analyst in a very concrete sensual way with her wet hands. This acting out was flanked by irritations, such as the fact that she was not sitting on the chair waiting, but was on the toilet, that she hesitated to shake my hand, etc. The fact that she had her faeces in her hands was a milestone. The fact that she had her excrement in her hands, smeared it on herself, ate it, had long been known to both of us, but these were words, words, words, as Prince Hamlet says (see also Freud, 1926e), empty shells conveying nothing sensual, let alone psychic. In this case, the communication that she held the excrement in her hands became a presentation spoken in an interpsychic space. The sensual was implemented almost forcibly – and I felt emotional reactions (disgust and inner distancing), with which I took refuge in expectable and explainable patterns on the one hand, but on the other hand began to suspect that something completely unknown was lurking here. I.e. a progredient movement towards a presentation that was sensualised in a regredient way.

Until the moment of presence, however, this material remained only presumed knowledge (K) about the world in which my patient lived, but was not understanding. An understanding only emerged at the moment of presence and subsequently also changed this preliminary knowledge. It has now taken on a psychic quality. We tend to experience the psychic quality that only appeared in the aftermath as if the psychic quality had also existed in the past.

This point is important because it underlines the treatment recommendations (see above). As long as the breakdown has not yet occurred in the relationship, our intuition is blind, it is necessary to formulate very close to the experience, to be careful with objectal and psychic dimensions. Otherwise we run the risk of understanding the liquid as tears in a person who seems to be crying, even qualifying it as mourning. Restraint is imposed on us because "hasty knowledge that could not be obliterated or corrected" can have "irreversible and unalterable consequences" (to paraphrase Bion's beautiful example; 1975, 49).

If we return to the patient whose mother was a drug addict, we can see how much a person who barely understands relationship, separation, i.e. facts of life, has adapted to the demands of the "normal" world, but at the core of his personality is probably still huddled under a duvet. In the analytical relationship, he dares to communicate that his girlfriend has broken up because of his depression. In everyday communication, the irritating barb ("because of my depression") would probably have gone unnoticed to avoid conversational complication. The patient has probably perfected his camouflage for years, disguising excessive demands. In his autistoid withdrawal, an object becomes dangerous, as it can tear open the second skin; in the hope of an object, there is the threat of expulsion, which also existentially threatens the self. The place under the duvet, however, is the permanent presence of catastrophe.

The moment of presence, in which her/his psychic disconnection with the world in which everything is extinguished, is a caesura. The female patient entered a suicidal whirlpool; the male patient entered a state of being torn away in a panic-psychotic way (fear of panic attack). How does it feel when suddenly the enveloping excitement is missing, how to suddenly be without a blanket? Like a burnt child, without skin, every draught of air hurts? Like a premature baby, still being intubated, not even able to cry out (the patient was silent, sitting up, because of the fear of a panic attack)? What of the "pre-psychic" non-existence will remain in the "post-psychic" existence, what will have really changed, what might seem like never having been?

Holding dominated the phase until the existential caesura. After the caesura, understanding and containing dominate, eventually paranoid-schizoid and depressive dynamics. In essence, however, we only have to do one thing: Be there and encounter…

Notes

1 Once, when I was stuck during disassembly, he noticed and just said: "Like this" (= this is how you have to do it) and showed me very briefly where I should place the screwdriver. For a tiny moment he looked at me and smiled – a smile like a psychic birth; it still touches me today.

2 Maria Rhode describes a touching sequence when a child with quite severe autistic disorder "one day, quite unusually, began to make the bird-like, chirruping sounds that babies begin to make at about 6 months, though he was turning his back to me as he did so. I was vividly reminded of how delighted my husband and I had been by these sounds when our eldest child had made them, decades earlier." Quite spontaneously, I commented, "Little baby bird noises." I was not expecting any kind of response, so I was floored when Mohammed said, in a normal voice and quite clearly, "Little baby bird noises." His tone made it clear that this was agreement rather than echolalia" (Rhode, 2023). From echolalia to an answer/agreement – a quantum leap!

3 Allen and Mendelson (2000) propose a treatment technique that requires such immersion in this distant world. They describe a treatment in which a mother enters her child's autistic world: Her child repeatedly makes a car crash into the wall. The mother sits down next to it, and does the same. Then the cars collide, and contact develops. Contact also develops because the mother "was" in the autistic world; her child felt accepted in its horror of the strange non-autistic world.

4 There could be connections here with the considerations of Ferrari and Lombardi. When the elements become extremely intense and decomposing as a result of the failure of the unfolding function, they lose their sensual function.

5 I think that Winnicott's and Bion's theory are not compatible, especially because of the underlying concept of object and that of "environment." However, since Winnicott's concept of object and environment in the self (infant) are to be thought of as an intrapsychic entity, I believe that important moments of Winnicott's "holding" can be integrated into a Freud-Bionian view.

6 In 2008 I described a case in which, also due to lack of experience, I had not succeeded in sublating the presence moment "well," but then failed mainly because of the patient's subsequent psychotic reaction, which I thought was a malignant regression and not a benign progression. The patient broke off the treatment but, when he came back again after a long time, was able to appreciate my "earnest effort," as if he had perceived my will to hold.

7 In my opinion, the dynamics of Nachträglichkeit always include both arrows of time, even though one forward or backward time vector may dominate. I will therefore not distinguish between deferred action and après coup in the following, but always use the German words nachträglich/Nachträglichkeit.

The concept of Nachträglichkeit is conceived temporally (see here Hock (2005, 293), who sees the diachronic temporal level suspended in the synchronic one and links Nachträglichkeit to the latter). Two vectors of time can be discerned in the case of Nachträglichkeit (see Freud, e.g., 1895; 1918b, 72; 1939a; Loch, 1988, 1993; Laplanche, 1992; Birksted-Breen, 2003, 2009; Hock, 2003, 2005; Eickhoff, 2005; Faimberg, 2005; Sodre, 2005; Dahl, 2010). In one, Nachträglichkeit follows the chronological arrow of time. In the other, Nachträglichkeit works against the chronological arrow of time. In one the present is interpreted in light of the past, in the other the past in light of the present, two time frames with a latency inserted. The dispute between deterministic and constructivist-consensual has long occupied psychoanalysis (e.g. the conflict between Loch, 1988, and Pasche, 1988; see Eickhoff, 2005). I am not an expert on the concept of Nachträglichkeit, but two objections seem to me worth considering: In my opinion, the reference system of psychoanalysis, the psychic, is missed in the question about a historical-objective determinacy. Historical, factual data do not belong to the psychic reference system. Furthermore, in the debates around Nachträglichkeit, the psychoanalyst is given primacy in interpreting the contexts. I do not share these positions either. See Nissen (2023); also Scarfone (2016).

8 Another example can be found in Zeitzschel (2023), who empathetically and comprehensibly describes a treatment in which nameless parts charge the dynamic processes.

9 It goes without saying that all the following treatment and theoretical considerations are retrospective. I never think in a session (my first sentence to any control analysand is: "Who thinks has lost").

10 Alvaraez (2004) emphasises the importance of this attunement in non-psychicised states in the broad sense.

11 Why Bion refers at this point to saturated concepts such as splitting, inhibition, etc. (see page 60), is not clear to me. Nor am I able to connect the idea of overcoming the caesura in a penetrating way with a method of communication (59) with his reflections on O.

12 I do not want the following to be understood as a discussion of the qualia problem, but rather as a clinical description of technical limits.

Chapter 5

Critical conclusion

5.1 Back to the beginning: on the determination of the nameless

Let us return to one of our initial questions: the subject and location of the nameless.

When Bion writes that we cannot interpret the "sights" that a foetus "sees," what does that mean? Can we intuit them? Or do we come up against an inescapable limit?

What does it mean when Freud writes that the psychic mother-object replaces the biological foetal situation for the child, that there were no objects in the intrauterine life (see above; 1926d)?

Can we recognise or at least intuit psychic structure and dynamics in an objectless state? Autoerotism, or primary narcissism, which Freud seems to equate in some writings,[1] are undifferentiated, indeed objectless states.

Reflection will quickly suggest that if any such fixation of the libido to the subject's own body and personality instead of to an object does occur, it cannot be an exceptional or a trivial event. On the contrary, it is probable that this narcissism is the universal and original state of things, from which object-love is only later developed, without the narcissism necessarily disappearing on that account (Freud 1916–17, 416).

Freud also makes important statements about the ego, or consciousness: "... we are bound to suppose that a unity comparable to the ego cannot exist in the individual from the start; the ego has to be developed. The auto-erotic instincts, however, are there from the very first;..." (1914c, 76–77). Later Freud paraphrases: "'... I am the breast.' Only later: 'I have it'..." (Freud, 1938b, 299).

I understand autoerotism/primary narcissism in two ways: It is an objectless, un-differentiated state without a developed ego, thus without systemic consciousness, an intrauterine state that persists after birth, in which the mother in her primary maternity maintains the illusion of a foetal situation temporarily-phasically. This state is necessary for digestion, thus also for the establishment of binocular functions; it exists unconsciously throughout life, "does not disappear." Such digestion is objectless, but, since the object establishes and replaces the "foetal situation," it is not objectless. The objectal secures the objectless state (even though the infant naturally has objectal capacities).

DOI: 10.4324/9781003434207-6

As the psychic apparatus develops and differentiates, objectless digestion becomes a function of the unrepressed unconscious. This function can then be directed towards all kinds of contents. But can we grasp it? Can it be intuited?

If we assume that the psychic can only arise and develop in a relationship and if we assume that we can only "analyse" the subjects that are common to the analytic couple, the answer can only be that this domain/this sphere remains closed to us. Bion emphasises this point again and again: only what is accessible to both the analyst and the patient can be investigated! Bion formulates it very harshly: Everything else can be left aside as irrelevant (e.g. 1965, 48–49; see also endnote Chapters 2, 7). Psychoanalysis can (at present) only make statements about the subject area that shows itself in the (transference) relationship. Only when the unrepressed unconscious, the unstructured unconscious, shows itself via descendants in the relationship can it be investigated. That is, if the function fails, the analysand will try to make the analyst to the object of the foetal situation, or enact that the holding object that ensures the objectless digestion is not there. Then we can get an inkling of such states in the relationship via the sensuality that runs along with it, i.e. we can see his sights of the world in a limited way.

But then we are no longer dealing with the unstructured unconscious, but with a "pathological unconscious." That is, the unrepressed unconscious that does not show itself in the relationship cannot be examined for its content. But if it does show itself in the relationship, it has become a pathogenic unconscious.

Psychoanalytic research can, however, make statements about the wider unconscious. We can infer functions, modes, ways of processing, etc., of the unconscious, i.e. displacement, condensation, no asymmetrical logic, timelessness, other dimensions/space, symmetrical logic, bi-logical structures, etc. Freud and Matte-Blanco have done this in an exemplary way. But psychoanalysis cannot influence these forms of processing; if we take Bion's great discovery, binocularity, seriously, it would even be wrong to strive for such influence. We can only try to guess at them, to describe them and to understand them as precisely as possible in order to draw conclusions for analytical practice.

The considerations on the unconscious make it very doubtful whether it makes sense to speak of one unconscious at all. Freud has described various characteristics of the unconscious, as already mentioned: primary process (mobility of occupations), timelessness and substitution of the external reality by the psychic one, displacement, condensation, no negation, non-contradiction, coexistence of contradictions and psychic states, no causality or causality as succession, simultaneity, etc. (see 1900a, 1915e). But with his model of topical, formal and temporal regression, Freud has de facto segmented the unconscious both horizontally and vertically. Matte-Blanco also attempted to describe unconscious orders with his fundamental distinction between asymmetrical and symmetrical logic. The bi-logical stratified structure with its specific strata and forms (e.g. Alassi, Simassi, Tridim) and infinity make it possible to assume different levels of unconsciousness. Freud and Matte-Blanco thus investigate the modes of functioning, processes, forms and mechanisms of the unconscious, which (can) act on the most diverse contents. Can psychoanalytic intervention, change be made in this field? I think not.

Only when these processes become dysfunctional, i.e. enter the relationship through content or disturbed functions, can psychoanalytic work be done. The shift from content to process proclaimed by many analysts may have its reason precisely in this: Dysfunctional processes lead to the disruption of unconscious processing, blocking binocular processing. The release of these processes can thus take precedence over the content – even if this release then becomes the content. It can make sense, for example, to work on the disturbance of the function of "objectless digestion" without looking for the exact "content" conditions.

But all these processes remain in the psychic-objectal, unconscious space and emerge when disturbances occur.

The situation is different with nameless states. One of the constitutional characteristics of the nameless is that they are objectless, or, more precisely, that hope (pre-conception) has been so severely damaged in the earliest stages of life that it has been abandoned, or if remnants still glimmer, the reactivation of hope is avoided. They become encapsulated and differentiated sensual qualities atrophy in pleasure/unpleasure, pleasure or pain, excitement or dullness. They are thus excluded from the central unconscious processings, no more clearly: They are excluded from almost all unconscious and preconscious/conscious processes. I.e. they are not to be located in the unrepressed or unstructured unconscious, they are not unconscious/conscious, they lie beyond the psychic. Therefore, it is necessary – as explained in detail – to slowly sensualise and psychicise them in holding, to finally let them be there via a moment of presence, so that they can become.

The fact that the nameless states do not disappear into the depths of the unconscious, but persist actually (even if perhaps only as a faint background noise almost completely withdrawn from attention), means that they can become the subject of analytical work.

5.2 On the criticism of Bion's terms

The criticism of Bion's terminology is not unfounded and massive. For one thing, he used many terms only temporarily (e.g. revêrie) and the implicit definitions do not meet scientific standards. But science is a living process – and the advance into new, unknown realms cannot take place with well-defined terminology. However – with his terms such as absolute truth, deity, etc., Bion himself has, in my opinion, contributed to the fact that the border to unscientificness has been crossed. Such concepts are valid in the field of mysticism and theology, not in that of scientific psychoanalysis.

But in addition to this fundamental criticism, there are also scientific decisions by Bion that have favoured the conceptual ambiguities. I would like to demonstrate this, in my opinion, necessary system-immanent critique on two important terms.

Bion writes that he finds the theory of the primary and secondary process insufficient, as it makes it necessary to assume two systems, whereas the α-function acts on all "emotional experiences," so that dreaming becomes possible in waking as well as in sleeping (see e.g. Bion, 1962, 54). He thus elevates the α-function to the sole variable in the psychic apparatus and its dynamics, which, if it is functional, has a transformative effect on all impressions that the personality has to process.

This, however, blurs all orders. The systems (in the first topical model) are fundamentally incompatibly *organised*. The Cs and Pcs systems, for example, are committed to the reality principle, the Ucs to the pleasure principle. Primary and secondary process, like pleasure and reality principle, are the functions that act on the events to be processed and produce completely different logics (psycho-logics), even though, as Matte-Blanco has shown, there can be bi-logical hybrids. This difference, according to my thesis, is what makes binocular processing possible in the first place, which knows a multitude of mechanisms in addition to dreams.

If everything is subordinated to one function (α-function), all forms of processing become blurred, the differences necessary for processing and structure formation fail, and differences (conscious unconscious; day-night; inside-outside) can no longer be used (it is interesting, as mentioned, that Bion does not want to distinguish between inner sensations and outer stimuli; see Bion, 1962, Chapter 2 para. 1).

Furthermore, it becomes problematic in my opinion that Bion's attempt to define the α-function implicitly has failed (as also evidenced by the multiple use by all authors; cf. also Bion's discussion of this approach: Introduction in "Learning from Experience"). An implicit definition needs an intuitively grasped and graspable subject that eludes explicit definition (a very nice example is Hilbert's Non-Euclidean Geometry). Freud chooses a completely different procedure: Concepts (e.g. reality testing) are formed from clinical empiricism, which are implicitly differentiated after their introduction.

Furthermore, it seems to me that Bion seems to almost completely neglect the horizontal and vertical differentiation of the unconscious system with its complicated dynamic interferences, which, as briefly shown, plays an important role in Freud and Matte-Blanco. Can this complexity really be captured with just one function? Don't very different functions and catalysts have to work in parallel and serially?

With the setting of the α-function as the sole mode of functioning and the failed implicit definition, it becomes clear in my opinion that it is difficult to differentiate between revêrie, α-function, dreaming, hallucination and also intuition; they ultimately lose their discriminatory power. Dream-work-α, on which some postbionians rely, will not remedy this, and will even increase the confusion.

The other concept that plays an important role in Bion's work from 1965 onwards is that of the infinite. For Bion in psychotic transformations the analyst

...has to deal with relationships of a domain that has no finite limitations. The terms psycho-analytic invariant, variable and parameter are meaningful in a universe of discourse that has in one important respect no realization corresponding to it; his interpretations have characteristics of relatedness that are applicable to his universe of discourse, but not to the phenomena they represent, since those phenomena possess a relatedness, if there is one, appropriate to an infinite universe.

(Bion, 1965, 44–45)

Unlike Freud, Bion focuses on finite and infinite: "The differentiating factor that I wish to introduce is not between conscious and unconscious, but between finite and infinite" (1965, 46).

But what is the "infinite" in Bion? He first associates it with the formless and the void (see also 1992, 308):

"The rising world of waters dark and deep

Won from the void and formless infinite." (Milton: Paradise Lost. in Bion, 1965, 151)

This wringing can only succeed through becoming: "I am not interpreting what Milton says but using it to represent O. The process of binding is a part of the procedure by which something is 'won from the void and formless infinite'; it is K and must be distinguished from the process by which O is 'become'. The sense of inside and outside, internal and external objects, introjection and projection, container and contained, all are associated with K" (1965, 151). And later Bion writes: "Evidently the impulse to achieve saturation is unlikely to be fulfilled because in addition to the limitations of human capacity there is the factor of 'the void and formless infinite' which, whether thought of as in the mind of man or outside it, cannot be known but must be 'become,' that is, saturated in a particular way" (1965, 155).

That is, the infinite is associated with O, or is identical with O, and cannot be grasped with K.

If one could still understand this view with the efforts to wrest something from the unconscious as void and formless infinite, Bion finally goes a step further and connects the infinite with the deity or the thing-in-itself, etc. (1970, 26), concepts which, as already mentioned, are not part of the analytical subject area.

In the post-Bionic literature, it is often associated with Matte-Blanco's concept of the infinite. However, Matte-Blanco's theory is based on set theory, from which he derives the concept of the infinite with reference to Dedekind (1998, 69). The principle of symmetry (1998, 52–54) shows itself in different strata; Matte-Blanco distinguishes six strata. The principle of symmetry is already very clear in the third and fourth strata. For example, in the third stratum (symmetrisation of the class), all objects of a set that have a characteristic in common are treated as if they were the same: All men with blue eyes not only have the characteristic "blue eyes" in common, but are identical as objects. In the fourth stratum (formation of wider classes which are symmetrised), objects of a set that have a feature in common are not only treated identically in the set, but equated with the superordinate set (wider class); men with blue eyes are thus identical with all men.

But if symmetry can be thought of this far, then Euclidean space is not sufficient (and vectorially ordered, chronological time cannot represent the processes). If the subset is equinumerous to the set, it is infinite, according to Dedekind's definition, to which Matte-Blanco refers: "a set is infinite if and only if fit can be put in bi-univocal correspondence (i.e. it is equinumerous) with a proper part of fit" (Matte-Blanco, 1998, 69). In the symmetric, *n*-dimensions are required.

According to Matte-Blanco, this creates the necessity for the psychic system to "break down" the *n*-dimensions for asymmetrical operating, i.e. to reduce them to the common dimensions. The conscious operates in Euclidean space and chronological times. An illustrative example of such reduction is that a triangle (two-dimensional) is to be mapped onto a line (one-dimensional). The ABC of the triangle, for example, becomes CABC (see Matte-Blanco, 1998, 87–88).

Most psychic states and dynamics are structured bi-logically, i.e. symmetrically-asymmetrically. Based on these set-theoretical considerations, Matte-Blanco designs a model of the unconscious and the psychic apparatus.

Questions arise for me: Can the unconscious really be grasped in terms of set theory? Can it be conceptualised as sets? I don't think so. The unconscious is far too dynamic, amorphous, impulsive, a cauldron full of seething energies in which the most diverse presentations, desires, etc., are sometimes boiled, sometimes fried, sometimes steamed, etc., sometimes cooked on a high flame, sometimes on the lowest economy flame, extremely oscillating, hardly lingering. Set theory is too static, orderly.

The transference of a mathematical theory into psychoanalysis has opened up important perspectives and had a catalytic effect. But in my opinion, a transplantation of such a theory (as well as other interdisciplinary attempts) is not possible.

Bion leaves his concept of the infinite dark and undefined, thus opening the door for the infinite to be filled with Matte-Blanco by some "postbionians." But would his concept of "Infinite" be compatible with Matte-Blanco? I don't think so – and it seems to me that Matte-Blanco would also be cautious here (see Matte-Blanco, 1983). Bion's void and formless infinite can hardly be conceived of as a set, but rather requires a constant willingness to encounter the unknown in such a way that it can happen. Matte-Blanco operates in K; Bion heads for O-becoming.

I wonder why Bion does not stick to his term "O," but instead introduces a term that he associates with O, but which carries with it more than a penumbra of associations. I see a great danger in this. For example, are states really infinite or total? There is a big difference. If everything is gripped by hate or love, is it infinite? Is it felt infinite? Or does it just take hold of everything, so is it total? What is this "everything"?

And aren't we in danger of confusing the indeterminacy of the psychic (not only the unconscious, but also the conscious! see presentative symbol) with infinity? If we cannot completely determine something, this does not mean that it is infinite.

Wittgenstein spoke of the fact that a "picture held us captive" (1984, §115). The concept of the infinite contains this danger. Wittgenstein recommends, in order to get out of this imprisonment, simply to look:

> Consider for example the proceedings that we call "games". I mean board-games, card-games, ball-games, Olympic games, and so on. What is common

to them all? – Don't say: "There must be something common, or they would not be called 'games'" – but look and see whether there is anything common to all. – For if you look at them you will not see something that is common to all, but similariries, relationships, and a whole series of them at that. To repeat: don't think, but look!

(1984, §66)

No memory, no desire, no understanding in philosophy.

5.3 From throwing away the ladder

Wittgenstein once again:

Meine Sätze erläutern dadurch, dass sie der, welcher mich versteht, am Ende als unsinnig erkennt, wenn er durch sie – auf ihnen – über sie hinausgestiegen ist. (Er muss sozusagen die Leiter wegwerfen, nachdem er auf ihr hinaufgestiegen ist.)

(Wittgernstein, 1922, Satz 6.54)

My propositions are elucidatory in this way: he who understands me finally recognizes them as senseless, when he has climbed out through them, on them, over them. (He must so to speak throw away the ladder, after he has climbed up on it.)

(Wittgernstein, 1922, Satz 6.54)

Do we have to throw away Bion's ladder? Has it done its job? Lombardi (but also others) seems to think so: "Today use of Bion's perspective would require, for example, a disappearance of his distinguishing language (grid, alfa, beta, caesura, and so on), for leaving place to current contemporary authors' new observations and new hypotheses" (Lombardi, 2022, 208).

Bion himself practised the temporary use of terms, simply dropping many again. So we should find the courage to ask: Do we still need these terms and sentences? (Wittgenstein does not speak of "needing" (brauchen), but of "senseless" (unsinnig) – thus using a word that is massive in terms of scientific theory: "unsinnig" (translated in English as "senseless" or "nonsensical"), which in German is at the same time ambiguous: meaningless, senseless, but also including the non-sensible.) What were Bion's terms good for? Almost all of Freud's terms exist, differently named, determined, more differentiated and theoretically justified...

From my point of view and understanding, Bion changed psychoanalysis permanently in two dimensions: With his reflections on projective identification and his theory of thinking, he has completely reweighted and placed at the centre the self the object and the relationship between them (also unlike Klein, for whom the object, formulated in a very template-like way, nevertheless remained an "object of observation"). Inseparable from these considerations is the theory of the binocular functioning of the conscious/preconscious and unconscious systems. When a child projects inner states that it cannot think into the mother and the mother returns them psychically digested and transformed, the aforementioned three central dimensions that Bion discovered are involved. This results in a new perspective on the self, the object, and the analytic couple, but also on relationship and groups. Everything that affects the psychic system is continuously processed binocularly, unconsciously as well as consciously/preconsciously. This indeed puts the processes in their place, in my view equally to the contents. In many disorders, it can be seen ad hoc that, for example, the unconscious does not or cannot do its "job" (to put it in a casual way). The simplest example: In every obsessive-compulsive disorder, it becomes obvious that the unconscious/preconscious perception and processing fails.

The irony of the story could be that Bion succeeded in this discovery because he radically reduced the complexity of psychic mechanisms, functions, modes, etc., with which Freud operated, and employed only one function, the α-function. This α-function operates in all systems and affects all sensations and impressions. If there is a function that operates in day and night thinking, in day and night dreaming, the binocular is already almost thought of. And if we take Freud's communication from Ucs to Ucs seriously, then in projective identifications the object can almost naturally be conceived as "digesting." If we now add to this the endless work imposed on every human child to understand the facts of life, separation, dependence, separateness, inside and outside, the Oedipal, in its never-resolvable paradox, etc., then the agony of learning to think (which Freud and Winnicott described similarly but differently) is clearly ad hoc. Much seems so self-evident today, no, too self-evident, that we run the risk of not fathoming the deep dimensions.

Bion's radical resetting of all terms, concepts, all certainties was necessary. Without this radicality, psychoanalysis would not be where it is today. But, do we still need Bion's "empty concepts"? No, I think we can safely put the ladder aside (but not throw it away!) and further differentiate the insights in the complexity of the psychic.

Let us close with a borrowing from Mozart's Magic Flute. Not three boys will be our guides, but with Freud and Bion we will limp on – which is no sin, as Freud noted.

Note

1 E.g. in 1916–17 and in 1915c. Differently, in his work "On Narcissism", Freud differentiates autoerotism and narcissism: "… there must be something added to auto-erotism – a new psychical action – in order to bring about narcissism" (1914c, 77). Nevertheless, I equate the terms in the following.

Bibliography

Abraham, K. (1916–17). Untersuchungen über die früheste prägenitale Entwicklungsstufe der Libido. In: *Ders.* (1971): *Psychoanalytische Studien.* 2 Bde. Hg. und eingeleitet von J. Cremerius. Frankfurt am Main: Fischer: 84–112.

Aguayo, J. (2018). D.W. Winnicott, Melanie Klein, and W.R. Bion: The controversy over the nature of the external object – Holding and container/ contained (1941–1967). *The Psychoanal. Q.*, 87(4):S.767–S.807.

Aisenstein, M. (2006). The indissociable unity of psyche and soma: A view from the Paris Psychosomatic School. *Int. J. Psychoanal.*, 87:667–680.

Alvarez, A. (1992). *Live company: Psychoanalytic psychotherapy with autistic, borderline, deprived and abused children.* London: Routledge. 256 p. [(2001). *Zum Leben Wiederfinden.* Frankfurt: Brandes und Aspel].

Alvarez, A. (2004). Finding the wavelength: Tools in communication with autism. *Infant Obs.*, 7(2–3):91–106. [(2006). Die Wellenlänge finden: Werkzeuge zur Kommunikation mit autistischen Kindern. In: Nissen B, editor. *Autistische Phänomene in psychoanalytischen Behandlungen* [Autistic phenomena in psychoanalytic treatments], pp. 55–72. Giessen: Psychosozial Verlag.]

Alvarez, A. (2012). *The thinking heart.* London and New York: Routledge.

Angeloch, D. (2021). The experience of the first world war in Wilfred Bion's autobiographical writings. *Psychoanal. Q.*, 90:1, 7–48.

Asseyer, H. (2002). The exclusion of the other. *Int. J. Psychoanal.*, 83:1291–1309.

Baranger, M., Baranger, W., & Mom, J.M. (1988). The infantile psychic trauma from us to Freud: Pure trauma, retroactivity and reconstruction. *Int. J. Psychoanal.*, 69:113–128.

Baron-Cohen, S. et al. (2000). *Understanding other minds. Perspectives from developmental cognitive neuroscience.* Oxford: Oxford University Press.

Barrows, K. (1999). Ghosts in the swamp: Some aspects of splitting and their relationships to parental losses. *Int. J. Psychoanal.*, 80:549–561.

Barrows, K. (ed) 2008. *Autism in childhood and autistic features in adults.* London: Karnac.

Barrows, P. (2001). The use of stories as autistic objects. *J. Child Psychother.*, 27:69–82.

Beland, H. (2012). Intregration eines „Über"-Ich. Die Beendigung einer sehr langen Analyse nach Anerkennung abgespaltener Über-Ich-Grausamkeit. In: B. Nissen, editor. *Wendepunkte. Zur Theorie und Klinik psychoanalytischer Veränderungsprozesse*, pp. 305–328. Giessen: Psychosozial-Verlag.

Benedetti, G. (1983). *Todeslandschaften der Seele.* Göttingen. Vandenhoeck & Ruprecht.

Bergson, H. (1927 [2013]). *Schöpferische Evolution.* Meiner Verlag: Hamburg.

Bergstein, A. (2013). Transcending the caesura: Reverie, dreaming and counter-dreaming. *Int. J. Psychoanal.*, 94:621–644.

Bergstein, A. (2014). Beyond the spectrum: Fear of breakdown, catastrophic change and the unrepressed unconscious. *Rivista Psicoanal.*, 60(4):847–868.

Bergstein, A. (2018). The psychotic part of the personality: Bion's expeditions into un-mapped mental life. *J. Amer. Psychoanal. Assn.*, 66(2):193–220.

Bergstein, A. (2020). Violent emotions and the violence of life. *Int. J. Psychoanal.*, 101:863–878.

Bergstein, A. (2022). Time and the unconscious. "Buried in the Future Which Has Not Happened". Unpubl. Paper.

Bick, E. (1968). The experience of the skin in early object-relations. *Int. J. Psychoanal.*, 49:484–486.

Bion, W.R. (1959). Attacks on linking. *Int. J. Psychoanal.*, 40:308–315.

Bion, W.R. (1962). *Learning from experience*. London: Tavistock.

Bion, W.R. (1962a). The psycho-analytic study of thinking. *Int. J. Psychoanal.*, 43:306–310.

Bion, W.R. (1963). *Elements of psycho-analysis*. London: Heinemann.

Bion, W.R. (1965). *Transformations*. London: William Heinemann.

Bion, W.R. (1967). Notes on memory and desire. In: J. Aguayo & B. Malin, editors. *Wilfred Bion: Los Angeles seminars and supervision*, pp. 136–138. London: Karnac, 2013.

Bion, W.R. (1970). *Attention and interpretation*. London: Tavistock.

Bion, W.R. (1975). Caesura. In: C. Mawson, editor. *The complete works of W.R. Bion*, vol. X, pp. 31–50. London: Karnac, 2014.

Bion, W.R. (1992). *Cogitations*. London: Karnac Books.

Birksted-Breen, D. (2003). Time and the après-coup. *Int. J. Psychoanal.*, 84:1501–1515.

Birksted-Breen, D. (2009). Reverberation time', dreaming and the capacity to dream. *IJP*, 90:35–51.

Blass, R.B. (2011). Introduction to "On the Value of 'Late Bion' to Analytic Theory and Practice." *Int. J. Psychoanal.*, 92:1081–1088.

Blass, R.B. (2012). "On Winnicott's Clinical Innovations in the Analysis of Adults": Intro-duction to a controversy. *Int. J. Psychoanal.*, 92:1439–1448.

Bohleber, W. (2000). Die Entwicklung der Traumatheorie in der Psychoanalyse. *Psyche – Z Psychoanal.*, 54(9–10):797–839.

Botella, C. (2014). On remembering: The notion of memory without recollection. *Int. J. Psychoanal.*, (95), 911–936.

Botella, C. & Botella, S. (2005). *The work of psychic figurability*, Weller A, translator, Par-sons M, preface. London: Brunner Routledge.

Botella, C. & Botella, S. (2013). Psychic figurability and unrepresented states. In: H.B. Levine, G.S. Reed & D. Scarfone, editors. *Unrepresented states and the construction of meaning*, pp. 95–121. London: Karnac/Int. Psychoanal. Assn.

Botella, S. (2005). L'Œdipe du ça ou Œdipe sans complexe. *Revue française de psychana-lyse*, 69:717–729.

Busch de Ahumada, L. & Ahumada, J.L. (2009). Autistische Mimesis im Medienzeitalter: Eine Fallgeschichte. In: B. Nissen, editor. *Die Entstehung des Seelischen. Psychoana-lytische Perspektiven*, pp. 141–163. Gießen: Psychosozial-Verlag.

Busch, F. (2018). Searching for the analyst's reveries. *Int. J. Psychoanal.*, 99(3):569–589.

Civitarese, G. (2015). Transformations in hallucinosis and the receptivity of the analyst. *Int. J. Psychoanal.*, 96(4):1091–1116.

Cohen, D. & Jay, S.M. (1996). Autistic barriers in the psychoanalysis of borderline adults. *Int J Psychoanal.*, 77:913–933.

Dahl, G. (2010). The two time vectors of Nachträglichkeit in the development of ego organization: Significance of the concept for the symbolization of nameless traumas and anxieties. *Int. J. Psychoanal.*, 91:727–744.

de Cesarei, A.O. (2005). Early trauma and narcissism–autism bipolarity. *Int. J. Psychoanal.*, 86:657–675.

de M'Uzan, M. (1977). Zur Psychologie der psychosomatisch Kranken. *Psyche*, 31(4):318–332.

Deutsch, H. (1926). Okkulte Vorgänge während der Psychoanalyse. *Imago*, 12:418–433.

Deutsch, H. (1934). Über einen typus der Pseudoaffektivität („als-ob"). *Int. Zeitschrift f. Psychoanalyse*, 20:323–335.

Eekhoff, J.K. (2023). Vorahnung: Hoffnung und Schrecken in der analytischen Stunde [Premonition: Hope and Dread in the Analytic Hour]. *Jahrb. Psychoanal.*, 87: 41–67.

Eickhoff, F.W. (2005). Über Nachträglichkeit. Die Modernität eines alten Konzepts. *Jahrb Psychoanal.*, 51:139–161.

Eshel, O. (2016). The "Voice" of breakdown: On facing the unbearable traumatic experience in psychoanalytic work. *Contemp. Psychoanal.*, 52(1):76–110.

Eshel, O. (2017). From extension to revolutionary change in clinical psychoanalysis: The radical influence of bion and Winnicott. *Psychoanal. Q.*, 86(4):753–794.

Faimberg, H. (2005). Après-coup. *Int. J. Psychoanal.*, 86:1 6.

Feldman, M. (1999). Projektive Identifizierung. Die Einbeziehung des Analytikers. *Psyche – Z Psychoanal.*, 53:991–1014.

Feldman, M. (2007). Spaltung und projektive Identifizierung. In: C. Frank & H. Weiß (Hrsg.). *Projektive Identifizierung*, pp. 27–46. Stuttgart: Klett-Cotta.

Ferrari, A R. (2004). *From the eclipse of the body to the dawn of thought.* London: Free Association Books.

Ferro, A. (2003). *Das bipersonale Feld.* Gießen: Psychosozial-Verlag.

Ferro, A. (2005). *Im analytischen Raum. Emotionen, Erzählungen, Transformationen.* Gießen: Psychosozial-Verlag.

Ferro, A. (2009a). *Transformations in dreaming and characters in the psychoanalytic field.* *Int. J. Psychoanal.*, 90(2):209–230.

Ferro, A. (2009b). Übertragung und Transformationen im Traum. In: B. Nissen editor. *Die Entstehung des Seelischen*, pp. 75–87. Gießen: Psychosozial-Verlag.

Fix Korbivcher, C. (2005). The theory of transformations and autistic states: Autistic transformations: A proposal. *Int. J. Psychoanal.*, 86:1595–1610.

Fix Korbivcher, C. (2014). Autistische Transformationen und das Verhältnis von container und contained. Wie man mit psychotischen und autistischen Phänomenen in Kontakt kommt. *Jahrbuch der Psychoanalyse*. Bd. 68. 89–105

Freud, A. (1968). Acting out. *Int. J. Psychoanal.*, 49:165–170.

Freud, S. (1895 [1950]). Project for a Scientific Psychology. SE Vol 1.

Freud, S. (1895). Studies on Hysteria. SE Vol 2.

Freud, S. (1900). The Interpretation of Dreams. SE Vol 4.

Freud, S. (1905a). Three Essays on the Theory of Sexuality. SE Vol 7.

Freud, S. (1910). The Future Prospects of Psycho-Analytic Therapy. SE Vol 11.

Freud, S. (1911b) Formulations on the Two Principles of Mental Functioning. S.E. 12.

Freud, S. (1911c). Formulations on the Two Principles of Mental Functioning. SE 12.

Freud, S. (1912a). Recommendations to Physicians Practising Psycho-Analysis. SE 12.

Freud, S. (1912b). The Dynamics of Transference. SE 12.

Freud, S. (1913i). The Disposition to Obsessional Neurosis, a Contribution to the Problem of the Choice of Neurosis. SE Vol 12

Freud, S. (1913c). On Beginning the Treatment (Further Recommendations on the Technique of Psycho-Analysis I). SE 12.

Freud, S. (1913j). The Claims of Psycho-Analysis to Scientific Interest. SE Vol 13.

Freud, S. (1914c). On Narcissism. SE Vol 14.

Freud, S. (1914g). Remembering, Repeating and Working-through (Further Recommendations on the Technique of Psycho-Analysis II). SE 12.

Freud, S. (1915c). Instincts and Their Vicissitudes. SE 14.

Freud, S. (1915d). Repression. SE Vol 14.

Freud, S. (1915e). The Unconscious. SE Vol 14.

Freud, S. (1916–17). Introductory Lectures on Psycho-Analysis. SE Vol 15–16.

Freud, S. (1917d). A Metapsychological Supplement to the Theory of Dreams. SE Vol 14.

Freud, S. (1917e). Mourning and Melancholia. SE Vol 14.

Freud, S. (1918b). From the History of an Infantile Neurosis. SE Vol 17.

Freud, S. (1920g). Beyond the Pleasure Principle. SE Vol 18.

Freud, S. (1923b). The Ego and the Id. SE Vol 19.

Freud, S. (1925a). A Note Upon the 'Mystic Writing-Pad'. SE 19

Freud, S. (1926d). Inhibitions, Symptoms and Anxiety. SE Vol 20.

Freud, S. (1926e). The Question of Lay Analysis. SE Vol 20.

Freud, S. (1927e). Fetishism. SE 21.

Freud, S. (1933a). New Introductory Lectures on Psychoanalysis. SE 12.

Freud, S. (1937c). Analysis Terminable and Interminable. SE Vol 23.

Freud, S. (1937d). Constructions in Analysis. SE 23.

Freud, S. (1938b). *Findings, Ideas, Problems*. SE Vol 23.

Freud, S. (1940a). An Outline of Psychoanalysis. SE 23.

Freud, S. (1940c [1938]). Splitting of the Ego in the Process of Defence. SE Vol 23.

Freud, S. (1940e). Splitting of the Ego in the Process of Defence. SE Vol 23.

Freud, S. (1980). Briefe. Hg. Von Ernst und Lucie Freud. S. Fischer Verlag. Frankfurt am Main.

Frith, U. (ed.) (1991). *Autism and Asperger syndrome*. Cambridge: CUP.

Gadamer, H-G. (1969/87). Über leere und erfüllte Zeit. In: Gesammelte Werke Bd. 4. Neuere Philosophie II. J.C.B. Mohr. Tübingen: Paul Siebeck Verlag, 137–152.

Gomberoff, M.J., Noemi, C.C., & Pualuan De Gomberoff, L. (1990). The autistic object: Its relationship with narcissism in the transference and countertransference of neurotic and borderline patients. *Int. J. Psychoanal.*, 71:249–259.

Green, A. (1975). The analyst, symbolization and absence in the analytic setting (On changes in analytic practice and analytic experience) – In memory of D. W. Winnicott. *Int. J. Psychoanal.*, 56:1–22.

Green, A. (2001). Todestrieb, negativer Narzißmus, Desobjektalisierungsfunktion. *Psyche*, 55(9–10):869–877.

Green, A. (2005 [1986]). The dead mother. In: *On private madness*, pp. 142–173. London, Taylor & Francis Group.

Green, A. (2009). Winnicott im Übergang zwischen Freud und Melanie Klein. *Jahrb. Psychoanal.*, 58:113–137.

Green, A. (2012). On construction in Freud's work. *Int. J. Psychoanal.*, 93(5):1238–1248.

Grotstein, J. (2004). The seventh servant the implications of a truth drive in Bion's theory of 'O'. *Int. J. Psychoanal.*, 85(5):1081–1101.

Grotstein, J. (2009). Dreaming as a 'curtain of illusion': Revisiting the 'royal road' with Bion as our guide. *Int. J. Psychoanal.*, 90(4):733–752.

Grotstein, J.S. (2007). *A beam of intense darkness. Wilfred Bion's legacy to psychoanalysis.* London, Karnac Books.

Heidegger, M. (1927). *Being and time*, J. Macquarrie & E. Robinson, translators. San Francisco, CA: HarperCollins, 1962.

Heimann, P. (1950). On counter-transference. *Int. J. Psychoanal.*, 31:81–84.

Heimann, P. (1960). Counter-transference. *British J. Med. Psychology.*, 33:9–15.

Hinshelwood, R.D. (2018): Intuition from beginning to end? Bion's clinical approaches. *Brit. J. Psychother.*, 34(2):198–213.

Hock, U. (2003). Zeit des Erinnerns. *Psyche*, 57:812–840.

Hock, U. (2005). Die Zeitlosigkeit des Unbewussten und die Wiederholung. In: K. Münch, et al, editors. *Zeit und Raum im psychoanalytischen Denken*, pp. 289–298. Frankfurt a.M: Tagungsband der DPV Frühjahrstagung.

Innes-Smith, J. (1987). Pre-oedipal identification and the cathexis of autistic objects in the aetiology of adult psychopathology. *Int. J. Psychoanal.*, 68:405–413.

Isaacs, S. (1948). The nature and function of phantasy. *Int. J. Psychoanal.*, 29:73–97.

Kahn, L. (2013). If one only knew *what* exists! In: H.B. Levine et al., *Unrepresented states and the construction of meaning. Clinical and theoretical contributions*, 122–151. London: Karnac Books.

Khan, M.M.R. (1963): Das kumulative Trauma. In: *Selbsterfahrung in der Therapie*, pp. 50–70. München (Kindler) 1977.

Kittler, E. (2022). Das Ringen um Darstellbarkeit – die Arbeit der Figurabiltät. *Psyche – Z Psychoanal.*, 76 (9/10): 914–944.

Klein, M. (1930). The importance of symbol formation in the development of the ego. In: *Love, guilt and reparation and other works*, pp. 219–232. London: Hogarth, 1975.

Klein, M. (1952). The origins of transference. *J. Psychoanal.*, 33:433–438.

Klein, S. (1980). Autistic phenomena in neurotic patients. *Int. J. Psychoanal.*, 61:395–402.

Klein, S. (1980/2006). Autistic phenomena in neurotic patients. *Int. J. Psychoanal.*, 61:395–402; In: B. Nissen, editor. *Autistische Phänomene in psychoanalytischen Behandlungen.* Giessen: Psychosozial-Verlag.

Klüwer, R. (1995). Agieren und Mitagieren – 10 Jahre später. *ZPTP*, 10:45–70.

Klüwer, R. (1997). Einblicke in die Welt des Autismus [Insights into the world of autism]. *Z Psychoanal. Theor. Prax*,12:151–165.

Klüwer, R. (2006). Der Ungeborene [The unborn] In: B. Nissen, editor. *Autistische Phänomene in psychoanalytischen Behandlungen* [Autistic phenomena in psychoanalytic treatments], pp. 169–188. Giessen: Psychosozial Verlag.

Krejci, E. (2012). Zur Verleugnung von Spaltungen in Übertragung/Gegenübertragung und zur „geheimen Verrücktheit" im analytischen Prozeß. In: B. Nissen, editor. *Wendpunkte. Zur Theorie und Klinik psychoanalytischer Veränderungsprozesse.* 163-190 Gießen: Psychosozial-Verlag.

Kris, E. (1956). The recovery of childhood memories in psychoanalysis. *Psa. Study Child*, 11:54–88.

Kütemeyer, M. (2003). Symptomdynamik hypochondrischer Beschwerden nach seelischem Trauma. In: Nissen, editor, S.251–S.266.

Langer, S.K. (1942). *Philosophy in a new key.* Cambridge, MA: Harvard University Press; London, England.

Laplanche, J. (1992). Die unvollendete kopernikanische Revolution in der Psychoanalyse. Frankfurt/M. (Fischer) 1996.

Laplanche, J. & Pontalis, J.B. (1972). *The languiage of psycho-analysis.* IPA Library.

Leikert, S. (2023). Die analytische Haltung und das körperliche Unbewusste – Bemerkungen zu einer behandlungstechnischen Kontroverse. *Jahrbuch der Psychoanalyse*, 86: 37–65.

Levine, H. (2023). Zur Genese der Deutung in einer sich verändernden Landschaft [On the Genesis of Interpretation in a Changing Landscape]. *Jahrbuch der Psychoanalyse*, Bd. 86: 77–98.

Levine, H.B. (2013). The colourless canvas: Representation, therapeutic action, and the creation of mind. In: Levine, H.B. et.al., editors. *Unrepresented states and the construction of meaning. Clinical and theoretical contributions*, 42–71 London: Karnac Books.

Levine, H.B. (2022). *Affect, representation and language. Between the silence and the cry.* London and New York: Routledge/IPA.

Levine, H.B. & Power, D.G. (eds) (2017). *Engaging primitive anxieties of the emerging self.* London: Karnac.

Levine, H.B., Reed, G. & Scarfone, D., eds. (2013). *Unrepresented states and the creation of meaning.* London: Karnac/IPA.

Loch, W. (1988). Rekonstruktionen, Konstruktionen, Interpretationen. Vom »Selbst-Ich« zum »Ich-Selbst«. *Jahrb. Psychoanal.*, 23, 37–81.

Loch, W. (1993). *Deutungs-Kunst. Dekonstruktion und Neuanfang im psychoanalytischen Prozeß.* Tübingen: edition discord.

Lombardi, R. (2022). Könnte eine Fokussierung auf den Körper, als primäres Objekt der Psyche, das Unzeitgemäße des kleinianischen Paradigmas überwinden? *Jahrbuch der Psychoanalyse*, 84:207–216.

Lombardi, R. (2009a). Symmetric frenzy and catastrophic change: A consideration of primitive mental states in the wake of Bion and Matte Blanco. *Int. J. Psychoanal.*, 90:529–549.

Lombardi, R. (2009b). Body, affect, thought: Reflections on the work of Matte Blanco and Ferrari. *Psychoanal. Q.*, 78:123–160.

Lombardi, R. (2016). *Formless infinity. Clinical explorations of Matte Blanco and Bion.* Transl. K. Christenfeld/G. Atkinson/A. Sabbadini/P. Slotkin. London: Routledge.

Lombardi, R. (2023). Übertragung auf den Körper und die Sprachregister der Analysesitzung. Kommentar zu Leikerts "Die analytische Haltung und das körperliche Unbewusste – Anmerkungen zu einer behandlungstechnischen Kontroverse". *Jahrbuch der Psychoanalyse*, 86: 67–75.

Luhmann, N. (1995). *Social systems*, Bednarz Jr J, Baecker D, translators. Stanford, CA: Stanford UP. 627 p. [(1987). *Soziale Systeme*. Frankfurt-am-Main: Suhrkamp.]

Madeleine, B., & Willy, B. (2008). The analytic situation as a dynamic field. *Int. J. Psychoanal.*, 89:795–826. [(1961–62). La situación analítica como campo dinámico. *Rev. Urug. Psicoanal.*, 4(1):3–54].

Marty, P., de M'Uzan, M. & Sellschopp-Rüppell, A. (1978). Das operative Denken („Pensée opératoire"). *Psyche*, 32(10):974–984.

Matte-Blanco, I. (1998). *Thinking, feeling, and being: Clinical reflections on the fundamental antinomy of human beings and world.* London: Routledge. New Library of Psychoanalysis, Hg. D. Tuckett, Bd. 5.

Meltzer, D. (1975a). The psychology of autistic states and of post-autistic states. In: D. Meltzer, J. Bremner, S. Hoxter, D. Weddell, & I. Wittenberg, editors. *Explorations in autism*, pp. 6–29. Strath Tay: Clunie.

Meltzer, D. (1975b). Dimensionality in mental functioning. In: D. Meltzer, J. Bremner, S. Hoxter, D. Weddell, & I. Wittenberg, editors. *Explorations in autism*, pp. 223–239. Strath Tay: Clunie.

Meltzer, D. (1975c). Adhesive identification. Contemp. Psychoanal., 11(3):289–310.

Meltzer, D., Bremner, J., Hoxter, S., Weddell, D., & Wittenberg, I. (1975). *Explorations in autism*. Strath Tay: Clunie Press.

M'Uzan, M. de (2020). Die Objektbeziehung. Zwischen wem, zwischen was? Für wen, für was? *Jahrbuch der Psychoanalyse*, Bd. 80: 159–179.

Miller, P. (2023). Bagatelle: Ein stiller transformativer Moment. *Jahrb. Psychoanal.*, 86:143–147.

Mitrani, J. (2009). Erstarrt im Schatten der Mutter. Zu den Nebenwirkungen der chronischen Verwendung auto-sensueller Schutzfaktoren. In: B. Nissen, editor. *Die Entstehung des Seelischen*, pp. 257–277. Giessen: Psychosozial-Verlag.

Mitrani, J. (2012). "Trying to enter the long black branches": Die Analyse autistischer Zustände im Erwachsenenalter. In: B. Nissen, editor. *Wendpunkte. Zur Theorie und Klinik psychoanalytischer Veränderungsprozesse*. Gießen: Psychosozial-Verlag.

Mitrani, J.L. & Mitrani, T. (eds) (2015). *Francis Tustin today*. London: Routlegde.

Moser, U. (2021). Kommentar zu Nissen: Das Erleben von Auflösung. *Jahrbuch der Psychoanalyse*, Bd. 82: 223-225

Nissen, B. (2000). Hpyochondria. A tentative approach. *Int. J. Psychoanal.*, 81:651–666.

Nissen, B. (2008). On the determination of autistoid organizations in non autistic adults. *Int. J. Psychoanal.*, 89:261–277.

Nissen, B. (2009). Die Geburt des Seelischen. Theoretische und behandlungstechnische Überlegungen zur autistoiden Dynamik am Beispiel einer Perversion. In: B. Nissen, editor. *Die Entstehung des Seelischen*, pp. 213–235 Giessen: Psycho-Sozial-Verlag.

Nissen, B. (2013). The scene in the psychoanalytic initial interview. *Rivista di Psycoanalisi*, LIX, 4:961–975.

Nissen, B. (2014a). Autistoide Organisationen. *Jahrbuch der Psychoanalyse*, Bd. 34: 56–73.

Nissen, B. (2014b). *Die Szene im psychoanalytischen Erstinterview*. texte. Psychoanalyse. Ästhetik. Kulturkritik. 34, Heft 4. 56-73 Wien: Passagen-Verlag.

Nissen, B. (2015a). Faith (F) and presence moment (O) in analytic processes: An example of a narcissistic disorder. *Int. J. Psychoanal.*, 96:1261–1281.

Nissen, B. (2015b). Zur psychoanalytischen Konzeptualisierung und Behandlung autistischer und autistoider Störungen. *Psychotherapeuten J.*, 14(2):100–119.

Nissen, B. (2015c). *Hypochondrie*. Gießen: Psychosozial Verlag.

Nissen, B. (2016). Melancholie und Zusammenbruch. Eine Neubetrachtung von Freuds „Trauer und Melancholie". *Jahrbuch der Psychoanalyse*, Bd. 73:123–146.

Nissen, B. (2018). Hypochondria as an actual neurosis. *Int. J. Psychoanal.*, 99:103–124.

Nissen, B. (2019). From word to deed. Why psychoanalysis needs laypersons. In: P.C. Sandler & G. Pacheco Costa, editors. *On Freud's "The Question of Lay Analysis"*, pp. 90–121. London: Routledge; New York.

Nissen, B. (2021a). Das Erleben von Auflösung. *Jahrbuch der Psychoanalyse*, Bd. 82: 217–221.

Nissen, B. (2021b). What is the psychic, how can it be grasped and understood? *Scand. Psychoanal. Rev.*, DOI: 10.1080/01062301.2021.1930505

Nissen, B. (2022). Kairos and Chronos. Clinical-psychoanalytical reflexions on 'Time'. EPF-Symposion on Time. Brussels, April 2022.

Nissen, B. (2023). Jenseits des Unbewussten? Kommentar zu Howard Levines Beitrag: "On the Genesis of Interpretation in a Changing Landscape". *Jahrbuch der Psychoanalyse*, Bd. 86: 99–108.

Nissen, B. (ed.) (2006). *Autistische Phänomene in psychoanalytischen Behandlungen*. Gießen: Psychosozial-Verlag.

Ogden, T.H. (1989). On the concept of an autistic–contiguous position. *Int. J. Psychoanal.*, 70:127–140.

Ogden, T.H. (1992). *The primitive edge of experience*. London: Maresfield Library.

Ogden, T.H. (1994). *Subjects of analysis*. London: Karnac.

Ogden, T.H. (2001). *Conversations at the frontier of dreaming*. Northvale/New Jersey/London: Aronson.

Ogden, T.H. (2004). The analytic third: Implications for psychoanalytic theory and technique. *Psychoanal. Q.*, 73:167–195.

Ogden, T.H. (2007). On talking-as-dreaming. *Int. J. Psychoanal.*, 88:575–589.

Ogden, T.H. (2015). Intuiting the truth of what's happening: On Bion's "Notes on Memory and Desire". *Psychoanal. Q.*, 84(2):285–306.

Power, D.G. & D. (2023). Intuition und at-one-ment: Ein klinisches Beispiel. (Intuition and At-one-ment: A Clinical Example). Erscheint in: *Jahrbuch der Psychoanalyse*, 87: 69–89.

Reik, T. (1932). Der Mut, nicht zu verstehen. *Psychoanalytische Bewegung*, 4:12–17.

Rhode, M. (1997). The voice as an autistic object. In: T. Mitrani & J.L. Mitrani, editors. *Encounters with autistic states*, pp. 41–61. Northvale, NJ: Aronson.

Rhode, M. (2018). Object relations approaches to autism. *Int. J. Psychoanal.*, 99(3):306–310.

Rhode, M. (2023). Auf Messers Schneide: Die Suche nach dem richtigen Abstand in der Arbeit mit Kindern aus dem Autismus-Spektrum. [On a knife-edge: Looking for the right distance in work with children on the autism spectrum]. *Jahrb. Psychoanal.*, 85: 17–35.

Rosenfeld, D. (1984). Hypochondriasis, somatic delusion and body scheme in psychoanalytic practice. *IJPA*, 63:311–319.

Rosenfeld, D. (2006). Autistische Abkapselung. In: B. Nissen, editors. *Autistische Phänomene in psychoanalytischen Behandlungen*, pp. 289–306 Giessen: Psychosozial-Verlag.

Rosenfeld, H. (1958). Some observations on the psychopathology of hypochondriacal states. *Int. J. Psychoanal.*, 39: 121–124.

Rosenfeld, H. (1964). *The psychopathology of hypochondriasis. In: Psychotic states*, H.A. Rosenfeld, editor. New York: International University Press, 1966.

Rosenfeld, H. (2004). Die Beziehung zwischen psychosomatischen Symptomen und latenten psychotischen Zuständen. *Jahrb. Psychoanal.*, 48:27–50.

Roussilion, R. (2015). Die Psychoanalyse des Narzissmus und die unvermeidliche "postmoderne" Psychoanalyse. Unpublished manuscript; DPV-Frühjahrstagung 2015.

Roussillon, R. (2021). Primäres Trauma, Spaltung und primäre, nichtsymbolische Bindung. *Zeitschrift für psychoanalytische Theorie und Praxis*, 36:189–216.

Sandler, P.C. (2005). *The language of Bion: A dictionary of concepts*. London: Karnac.

Sandler, P.C. (2009). *A clinical application of Bion's concepts*, vol. 1: *Dreaming, transformations, containment and change*. London: Karnac.

Sandler, P.C. (2018). Wirkliches Psychoanalyse ist wirkliches Leben. *Jahrbuch der Psychoanalyse*, 76: 125–164.

Sandler, P.C., et al. (1973). *The patient and the analyst. The basis of the psychoanalytic process*. London: G. Allen & Unwich.

Scarfone, D. (2016). Enactive cognition, the unconscious, and time. *Psychoanal. Inq.*, 36(5):388–397.

Schellekes, A. (2017). "Day-dreaming and hypochondria: When day-dreaming goes wrong and hypochondria becomes an autistic retreat." In: H.B. Levine, & D.G. Power, editors. *Engaging primitive anxieties of the emerging self: The legacy of Frances Tustin*, pp. 21–42. London: Karnac.

Schneider, G. (2006a). Der autistischer Kernbereich einer Borderline-Störung und die Entwicklung eines inneren Raums. [The autistic nuclear area in a borderline disorder and the development of an internal space]. In: B. Nissen, editor. *Autistische Phänomene in psychoanalytischen Behandlungen* [Autistic phenomena in psychoanalytic treatments], pp. 189–224. Giessen: Psychosozial Verlag.

Schneider, G. (2006b). Ein» »»unmöglichen« Beruf« (Freud) – zur aporetischen Grundlegung der psychoanalytischen Behandlungstechnik und ihrer Entwicklung. *Psyche – Z Psychoanal.*, 60:900–931.

Schneider, G. (2007). Ein»»unmöglichen« Beruf« (Freud) – das aporetische Prinzip in der Reflexion der psychoanalytischen Behandlungstechnik. *Psyche – Z Psychoanal.*, 61:657–685.

Schneider, G. (2014). Es gibt nicht das Wahre im Unwahren, wohl aber das Richtige im Falschen. *Jahrb. Psychoanal.*, 69:15–47.

Schütze, F. (1982). Narrative Repräsentation kollektiver Schicksalsbetroffenheit. In: E. Lämmert, editor. *Erzählforschung*, pp. 568–590. Metzler: Stuttgart.

Sodré, I. (2005). 'As I was walking down the stair, I saw a concept which wasn't there'. Or, après-coup: A missing concept? *Int. J. Psychoanal.*, 86:7–10.

Stern, D.N. (2004). *The present moment in psychotherapy and in every day life*. New York: W.W. Norton&Company.

Strachey, J. (1934). The nature of the therapeutic action of psycho-analysis. *Int. J. Psychoanal.*, 15:127–159.

Strauss, V. (2006). „Das unerbittliche Gedächtnis" ['The unrelenting memory']. In: B. Nissen, editor. *Autistische Phänomene in psychoanalytischen Behandlungen* [Autistic phenomena in psychoanalytic treatments], pp. 265–288. Giessen: Psychosozial Verlag.

Strauss, V. (2014). Vom Pilotfisch zur Analytikerin… Das Auftrennen der Naht. *Jahrbuch der Psychoanalyse*. Bd. 68: 107–135.

Tustin, F. (1972). *Autism and childhood psychosis*. Hogarth/New York: Jason Aronson, 1973.

Tustin, F. (1980). Autistic objects. *Int. Rev. Psychoanal.*, 7:27–39.

Tustin, F. (1981). *Autistic states in children*. Henley-on-Thames: Routledge & Kegan Paul.

Tustin, F. (1984). Autistic shapes. *Int. Rev. Psychoanal.*, 11:279–290.

Tustin, F. (1986). Autistic barriers in neurotic patients. New Haven, CT/Karnac: Yale University Press, produced by Free Association Books, 1987.

Tustin, F. (1988). The 'black hole'. *Free Assoc.*, 1:35–50.

Vermote, R. (2013). The undifferentiated zone of psychic functioning: An integrative approach and clinical implications. *Bulletin EPF*, 67:16–27.

Vermote, R. (2022). Übertragung-Gegenübertragung aus einer bionianischen Perspektive. *Jahrb. Psychoanal.*, 84:119–140.

Winnicott, D. (1960). The theory of the parent-infant relationship. *Int. J. Psychoanal.*, 41:585–595.

Winnicott, D. (1965). *The maturational process and the facilitating environment: Studies on the theory of emotional development*. Hogarth: Institute of Psycho-Analysis.

Winnicott, D.W. (1963). 'The mentally ill in your caseload'. In: *The maturational process and the facilitating environment: Studies on the theory of emotional development*. Hogarth: Institute of Psycho-Analysis, 1965, pp. 217–229.

Winnicott, D.W. (1969). The use of an object. *Int. J. Psychoanal.*, 50:711–716.

Winnicott, D.W. (1974). Fear of breakdown. *Int. Rev. Psychoanal.*, 1:S.103–S.107.

Winnicott, D.W. (1975). Through paediatrics to psycho-analysis, Chapter XXIV. *Primary Maternal Preoccupation* [1956]: 300–305.

Winnicott, D.W. (1975 [1956]). Primary maternal preoccupation. *Int. Psychoanal. Lib.*, 100:300–305. Chapter XXIV.

Wittgenstein, L. (1963). *Tractatus logico Philosophicus*. Frankfurt a.M.: Suhrkamp Verlag (SV).

Wittgenstein, L. (1984). *Philosophische Untersuchungen*. Frankfurt a.M. Werkausgabe in 8 Bänden STW.

Zeitzschel, U. (2017). Riccardo Lombardis Formless Infinity: Der Körper als Kompass. *Jahrbuch der Psychoanalyse*, 75:183–194.

Zeitzschel, U. (2018). Frühe Erfahrungen als Einstieg in die psychoanalytische Welt – Beobachterin und Seminargruppe in der analytischen Säuglingsbeobachtung. *Jahrb. Psychoanal.*, 77. Stuttgart: frommann-holzboog, 123–145.

Zeitzschel, U. (2019). *Zusammenbrüche des frühen Erlebens – Überlegungen zu einem psychoanalytsichen Deutungsprozess*. Unveröff. Manuskript.

Zeitzschel, U. (2022). Was können wir von Babys lernen? Die analytische Säuglingsbeobachtung als wünschenswerter Bestandteil der psychoanalytischen Ausbildung. *Kinderanalyse*, Heft 2. Stuttgart: Klett-Cotta Verlag, pp. 176–191.

Index

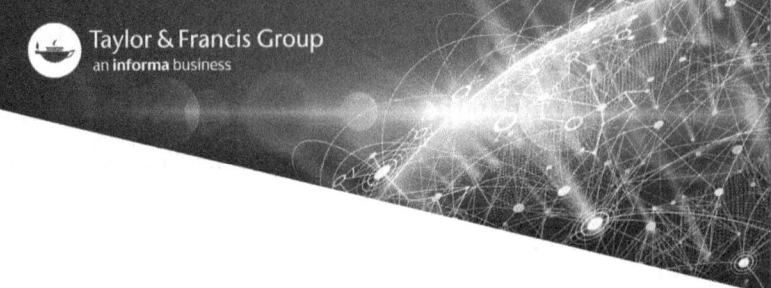
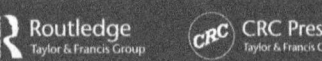